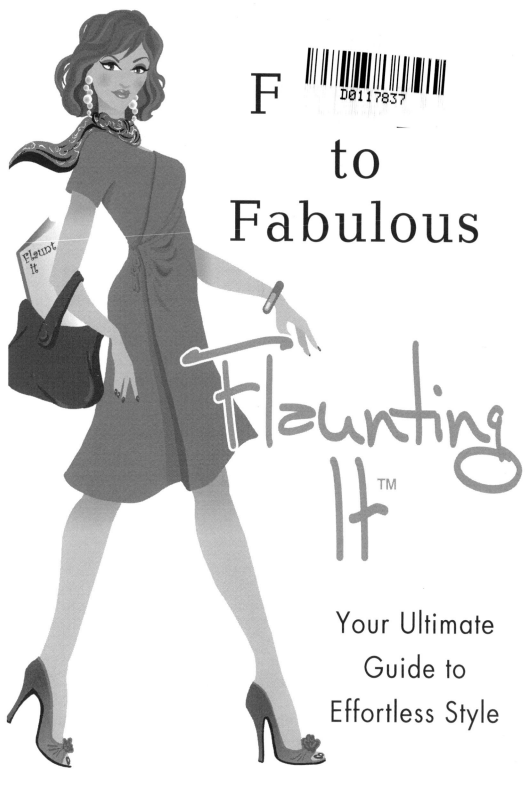

F
to
Fabulous

Flaunting It™

Your Ultimate
Guide to
Effortless Style

NATALIE JOBITY

Frumpy to Fabulous: Flaunting It™
Your Ultimate Guide to Effortless Style: Revised Edition

Copyright © 2010/2011 Natalie Jobity

Elan Image Management, LLC
PO Box 2695
Columbia MD 21045

Interior/Cover Design: Carolyn Sheltraw

Cover illustration: Maryam Hassanahmad

Back cover/back page photo credit: Kenneth Clapp Photography

Interior Illustrations: Ann-Cathrine Loo, a Swedish artist who has illustrated numerous books published in USA, United Kingdom, and Sweden.

ISBN -13: 9780982929704
ISBN-10: 0982929706

Printed in the United States by CreateSpace. Published by Elan Image Management, LLC

For information about special discounts for bulk purchases, please contact Elan Image Management LLC at Info@Elanimagemanagement.com

Note: This book includes the author's opinions and professional experience based on her work as an image consultant. The opinions and viewpoints on the brands/companies mentioned in the book are those of the author and they were made without payment or the expectation of payment from these companies. As of the completion of this manuscript in July 2010, and its revision in September 2011, the author was not a representative, affiliate, spokesperson or employee of any of the brands or companies mentioned in this book. The author and Elan Image Management LLC do not assume any liability of any kind for the purchase, use or trials of these brands or products and are not responsible for the performance of these products.

This book is dedicated to my late father, who encouraged me to see my own imperfect perfection; my Mother who by example, gave me my keen fashion, creative and aesthetic sensibilities; and to all the women just bursting to let their magnificence shine from the inside out.

– Natalie Jobity

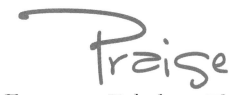

Praise

for *Frumpy to Fabulous: Flaunting It.*
Your Ultimate Guide to Effortless Style

"Finally, a practical book of tips for releasing your innate beauty - from the inside out. Natalie Jobity becomes your own personal image consultant in these pages - like getting $2,000 worth of image consulting for the price of a book! I am one of Ms. Jobity's clients, and I deeply appreciate her focus on inner as well as outer beauty. This book is a must read for sprucing up your appearance - and therefore increasing your ability to accomplish your goals. This is a book you'll cherish and refer to over and over again."
— Dr. Clare Albright, Psychologist and author of, *Neurofeedback: Transforming Your Life with Brain Biofeedback*

"Wow! "Frumpy to Fabulous: Flaunting It. Your Ultimate Guide to Effortless Style" is every woman's guide to learning how to look, live and feel her best through image. Women across the country are always searching for the secrets of the trade to looking good. As a personal strategist to thousands of mothers, women often share with me that they have forgotten or no longer know how to look their best. Moms especially stop shopping for themselves and forget what looks great on them. Now, we have an easy to read, funny and informative book that will give us the same advice of the stars' personal stylist. Natalie knows how to reach women of all sizes, shapes and color and has wowed thousands through her media appearances, wardrobe boot camps and image consulting services. This terrific book allows us to take Natalie home with us so we can take a view inside our closets and follow her turn-key system for anyone to go from Frumpy to Fabulous with a bit of effort. Thanks for giving moms the tools for looking fabulous and the permission to Flaunt it."
— Mia Redrick, The Mom Strategist. www.findingdefinitions.com

"If you've ever kicked yourself for looking dowdy when opportunity knocked or been less than impressed with the contents of your closet, after some tutoring from the knowledgeable Natalie Jobity, you'll be transformed into one of those women you pass in the street who look their fabulous best! "Frumpy to Fabulous: Flaunting It. Your Ultimate Guide to Effortless Style" will help you align how you feel on the inside with how you wish you looked on the outside, so you'll look better, be treated better, and exude confidence. Whether you're angling for a promotion, looking for a date, interviewing for a new job, or wanting to be a strong role model, it's imperative in our image-driven society that you look consistently polished, pulled together, and credible. Let Natalie show you how to become fabulous...and flaunt it!"
— Lesley Scott, Fashion Critic & Editor in Chief, Fashiontribes.com (a Top 10 Fashion Blog)

Note to Readers

Many women share stories similar to the anecdotes shared in this book. As I've worked with women over the years, their stories and challenges became recurring themes. The transformation anecdotes shared in this book, while inspired by these women, are fictional. They are illustrative of my work collectively and do not represent my work with one particular client. Any similarities to a particular woman in any way are purely coincidental and unintentional.

– Natalie

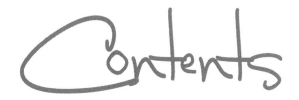

"Our deepest fear is not that we are inadequate. Our deepest fear is that we are powerful beyond measure. It's our Light not our darkness that most frightens us. We ask ourselves, who am I to be brilliant, gorgeous, talented, fabulous? Actually, who are you not to be...your playing small does not serve the world. There is nothing enlightened about shrinking so that others won't feel insecure around you...As we let our own light shine, we unconsciously give other people permission to do the same."

– Marianne Williamson, Return to Love

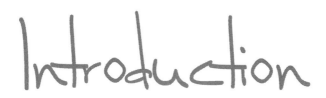

Introduction

Have you been Flaunting It?

If I told you looking fabulous isn't really as hard as it seems, would you believe me? You should. I wrote this book to show you how easy it can be to look and feel great once you are armed with information and empowered to dress with intent.

Intent?

Absolutely! Do you think fabulous women just walk out the door fabulous? Well, maybe a lucky few do. But most "fabulistas" you admire have put thought and effort into the way they look. They do so consistently, knowing that they reap social and professional benefits galore from being seen as women who dress well.

Well, guess what? You can too. I will show you how, with a little thought, effort and strategy, you can Flaunt your new image to the world, feeling and looking fabulous along the way, while gaining all the benefits your new stunning image entitles you to.

As a practicing image consultant, I work with women just like you, with similar life and body challenges, lack of expertise and knowledge, who desire to look great. I help women find their unique signature styles, encourage them to embrace their bodies and learn how to dress with an eye for figure flattery. I have observed that once women understand the art of dressing well and give themselves permission to dare to think they can aspire to look like their personal fashion icons, they become transformed. In a desire to share my expertise and secrets with women the world over, so they too can experience their own image transformations, this book was birthed.

When I use the words "frumpy" and "fabulous" in the title and within these pages, don't get hung up on the words. One woman's frumpy is another woman's best effort at looking good. It's all so relative. Similarly, don't let the word "fabulous" intimidate you. Fabulous is whatever your highest, finest vision of yourself is. It could be looking polished and pulled together—a goal for many women I work with. Or it could be achieving the heights of red carpet glamour. The notion of looking fabulous is unique to each woman, as will your journey on your path to fabulous.

I am here to arm you with the tools and the information, regardless of the end point of your journey. But know this: once you are really ready to put yourself out there and flaunt your fabulousness, you will be transformed along the way. It can be subtle or dramatic but it will happen if you are sincere in your desire for change.

BRINGING OUT YOUR UNIQUE BRILLIANCE

You have the power to choose how you show up. Are you choosing invisibility or radiating your full brilliance? Just as roses need sunlight and water to fully bloom, what brings out your brightest, finest, most brilliant bloom? Do you even know?

I believe all women really want to shine. They really do. But there are so many reasons why for some women, the glow emitted can be dull or non-existent: the dread of being judged; the unwillingness to own their own brilliance; poor information about how to enhance their God given beauty; a lack of confidence; poor self-esteem; bad habit; or just plain laziness. But mostly I've found for many women it ultimately boils down to fear: the fear of being vulnerable enough to expose who they really are. Because of fear these women may:

- Choose to be invisible

- Conform so they look like everyone else around them

- Make half-hearted efforts to look good, but don't follow through

- Make no effort at all

- Make an effort but become so self-conscious, they sabotage the effort

I wrote this book to empower, enlighten and inspire. I share anecdotes so you the reader can relate to different situations and know you are not alone in your fears, challenges and concerns. I want you to be emboldened to look and express exactly who you are, so that you are a true reflection of your inner beauty.

Looking good becomes second nature when you make it a habit. A habit becomes "a habit" by repeated behavior. If you only make the effort on special occasions, when your mother-in-law visits, when you go on a date, when you want to impress so and so, or any other selective occasion, the habit won't stick. You'll be back in your lackluster clothes in a heartbeat.

Your new intention has to come from a true desire to change the way you look. Yes, it's going to take lots of effort at first, but then before you know it, just like riding a bicycle, you'll soon forget you have those training wheels on, and all of a sudden you'll notice you are Flaunting It on a consistent basis.

When you *really* see yourself looking fabulous and amazing and are comfortable with what that looks like for you, invisibility, frumpy, blah, or dowdy are simply not options anymore. Not options. Looking great will become non-negotiable.

Do you realize the power in that statement? Flaunting is an attitude, a feeling, an energy, an air of utmost confidence that leaves everyone around you inspired. It is not about being a "Diva" (the negative connotations of that word), a fashionista, a show off, or an attention seeker. It is ALL about being comfortable in who you are and how you choose to express yourself. It's about being authentic, transparent and unapologetic. It's so about you and not about them.

It is truly liberating to have the self-assurance to show up as your finest expression in every moment. The deeper message woven into this book is about self-love, self-acceptance and self-expression. Ultimately, being Fabulous and Flaunting It is about letting your guard down so others get to see you in your full glory.

Seems so simple, right? So why aren't we Flaunting It all the time? Because putting yourself out there exposed to judgment and opinion, is hard. It is harder still when that self-expression goes against the grain. It is easier to take the safe, conformist path; to resist the urge to buckle against the norm.

But wait! This is a book about style, wardrobe and image. Why are we talking about self-acceptance and journeys? Because at the heart of it all is the mental game—the mind that brings up your insecurities, perceived flaws, imperfections, and self-esteem issues. The mind that can be the saboteur of every noble, good intention you have, image or otherwise. If you don't tackle your mind and the many ways it can repress your intentions, it is hard to realize a change from Frumpy to Fabulous. This is why I devoted a chapter in this book on tackling "image saboteurs".

You likely picked up this book to learn how to enhance the way you look, to achieve effortless style or perhaps to gain the knowledge so you have the confidence to Flaunt It. Yes! This book will equip you with all the knowledge, insider secrets, tips, tricks and whatnot, so you know what to wear and how to wear it to showcase the best of you. You have my word that after reading this book you will not only be more informed and educated about how you can apply tactics to look amazing, but more importantly, you will be motivated and inspired to implement them.

It is my mission to help elevate, liberate and inspire women to look their best regardless of the occasion. I believe it is my divinely appointed purpose to reveal to women how uniquely beautiful we all are. My unique life path and my life experiences to date —especially the really tough ones—make me a relatable champion for women and their image transformations. I keep it real. But that honesty comes from the deepest wells of compassion for women who struggle with their look. My voice in this book is that of an expert, yes, but it is also that of a trusted friend, a champion for you.

So many women who read this book over the past year have shared the wonderful ways this book has empowered them to change. It is always humbling to hear their stories and I am filled with gratitude that I can be a vessel for change and overjoyed that I made a difference.

What fulfills me? Making that difference. Being the catalyst for change. Seeing a woman transform from frumpy to (her) fabulous, seemingly overnight. Knowing that there are many thousands more like her for whom this book has ignited a spark or fanned a full flame of self-expressive fabulousness.

MY JOURNEY TO FLAUNTING IT

I have had many evolutions in my journey to Flaunting It. I was always acutely aware of the effect of clothing on my tall, lean frame growing up. I had to wear mandatory uniforms from elementary to high school that did nothing to flatter me. I did not feel attractive, to say the least. For much of my young life, growing up on the island of Trinidad & Tobago, it was truly difficult to find clothing to fit me. With my Mother's assistance, I had to live with being resourceful; getting clothing custom made for special occasions (a real treat!), attempting to make off the rack clothing work, and even sewing extra fabric on the edge of my favorite jeans as I grew too tall for them.

So much of the time I was trying to blend in as best as I could. I towered over all my peers from age 11. All of a sudden I had a growth spurt and I was 5' 9". By the time I was 13, I was 5' 11". I felt awkward and unattractive. I was so physically obvious and I didn't want to be. I often envied the petite girls whom the young boys seem to favor. They were so cute. And I was just klutzy and lanky. I disliked being so tall. I truly felt like a freak. By the age of 14, I was just a couple inches shy of my Dad who was a tall, strong, handsome man. I had grown to my full height of 6'1", and resented every second of it.

In spite of this internal struggle, I had a burgeoning sense of… style? At least I started to have strong opinions about how I wanted to look and clear role models I aspired to emulate. I devoured the teen magazines and even my Mother's "Glamour" and "Reader's Digest", to try to make sense of what could work for my body. The messages I got repeatedly growing up in my culture was that I needed more 'meat on my bones', that I needed curves, that my linearity was not attractive. It was encouraging that within these magazines, tall, thin girls were adored. There was a bigger world out there where models whose bodies looked more like mine were beautiful and revered. There was hope.

I cared so much about the way I looked, that I saved my weekly allowance for treasured pieces of clothing—a blue/white crinkle cotton shirt that caught my fancy, an ivory knit top, a pair of chino slacks that actually came to my ankles. Looking back I didn't always get it right. But I sure never gave up trying.

I remember my parents taking me on a shopping trip when I was 16 or so and being able to buy whatever I wanted. And I remember exactly what I picked out: a tiered red and white diagonal striped cotton mini skirt and a red and white striped top. I think that was the first short skirt I ever owned. I was thrilled with my bounty. I paired the two pieces together to go to a party and from the reaction of my peers and someone joking I looked like a candy striper, I'm pretty sure I didn't knock it out of the ball park. But I remember *feeling* so girly and pretty! And that's all that mattered.

It was at that time in my life that I really started to work with my height and understand the gift of being statuesque. I learned how to wear my hair and apply makeup to bring out the best of my features. My family took vacations abroad and I would come back with my suitcase full of new clothes that made me feel stylish. This was the 80's, so baggy pants and "Flashdance" inspired cut off tops were hip and flattered my frame. I went crazy for colors. And I absolutely fell in love with accessories: earrings, bangles, necklaces, belts, oh my!

By the time I went off to college in the United States at Rutgers University, I would have been considered trendy…with a definitive Natalie vibe developing. So much so that even as a freshman, I would often get stopped by other students who wondered if I was, get this, a model. A model!

College for me was truly a time of coming into my own, and gaining the self-esteem and confidence I lacked as a young girl. I was able to express myself through my appearance and it felt freakin' fabulous! I definitely loved it and I was Flaunting It.

That was so many years ago. What is significant is that, like everything else in life, there are cycles: cycles of growth, reinvention, rebirth and growth again. Youth is a time of self-expression and self-awareness. Adulthood brings its own challenges, which gives one pause and often requires one to begin anew.

One of my greatest challenges as an adult was truly "owning" my presence. By now, I had accepted my statuesque height. But acceptance isn't the same as reveling in it, is it? Beginning to understand the power in my presence and the beauty of shining in my full brilliance came to me from practicing yoga. There is a core pose that is the foundation of many standing yoga poses: Tadasana, also known as Mountain pose. At first blush, it just looks like a pose where you stand straight and tall. But it is so much more than THAT. As a yoga student, I found myself resisting this pose for years and not understanding why. I felt exposed and vulnerable in the pose and it made me so uncomfortable I had to fight the urge to cower inward every time.

One year on vacation, I decided to practice walking in Tadasana on the beach. I love everything about the ocean and I'm most relaxed around water. So I plugged my Ipod in my ears and started walking up and down the stretch of beach, walking in Tadasana. It was just for fun at first—I walked up and down and at some point even found myself sashaying to the music and the rhythm of the waves as they broke on the shore. At some point though, something magical started to happen. I started to *feel* my own power. Suddenly, I found myself walking faster and with each stride I could literally feel myself inching taller and taller towards the clear blue sky—from *inside* of me. I was now in full strut mode, and in my heart, in that moment, I knew I was unstoppable. Everything around me became a blur and all I became aware of was my exquisite presence, power and strength, out there on that beach. I felt as if I could just step out onto the water and walk on it. It was an incredible and unforgettable experience. It forever changed my understanding of the inner strength that always resides within us all.

From that moment on, I was no longer scared to stand in Tadasana in my yoga class—to embrace my full height, to keep reaching up from the crown of my head as I anchored my feet deeply into the floor, (hip distance apart), shoulders relaxed, pelvis tucked in, head facing forward and my body fully aligned. I finally got it. Standing in Tadasana isn't just about good posture. It is about owning your own power and feeling your strength as the Universe supports you. It is about being open, present and conscious to the magnificence that is you. It is about being fearless. It's about having the presence of a Mountain! What an awesome lesson and one of many that I learned from the practice of yoga.

I now love my height. It becomes me and I revel in it. I can't imagine having it any other way. But for so many years I resisted my body—I felt it was the enemy. The grass is always greener, isn't it? Thin girls want to be curvy, curvy girls want to be thin, and it goes on. We are never satisfied with who we are and what we have.

Someone wise said to me recently that the true strength and power within us comes from our 'essence'. It is no coincidence then, that throughout this book I try to underscore the importance of expressing your authentic self. My fabulousness and your fabulousness may look completely different, but at the end of the day we're both fabulous! I am here to guide you and share with you what I know, but it is you who must define for yourself your parameters for looking your best.

My style journey has had many incarnations and I expect I have a few left to go. But at this time in my life, I feel I have struck the perfect harmony between self-expression and restraint, seasoned yet playful, ladylike but alluring. My style now is a combination of my experiences, my lifestyle and my preferences as a woman in today's culture.

An important message I want you to understand as you read this book, is to learn to embrace who you are, what you look like, where you are right now. You can strive to lose weight, get fit, be healthy, firm up, et cetera. It is all good. But don't miss out on this present moment, the beauty that is within and of you right now. Learn to dress to flatter your body's unique lines and curves, not the body you wish you had. I now have the expertise to know what works for me and brings out my unique sparkle. It is my hope that after reading this book, you begin to tap into yours.

WHAT'S NEW IN THE REVISED EDITION?

In this revised edition, in addition to tweaking and updating content throughout the book, I've updated many of the illustrations from the original edition and added new ones as well. It is said that a picture is worth a thousand words and that seeing is believing. With that in mind, I wanted the illustrations to really come to life so that they inspire you. I've been inspired just by conceptualizing them.

In addition to sharing a little more of my journey in this introduction, and really setting the stage for the pages that follow, I added a whole new meaty chapter focused on what you wear to work. We spend so much time at work, yet so many women struggle with what to wear. I want you Flaunting It at the office as well! So Chapter 9 is brand new for this edition and it covers a lot of ground on the topic of appropriate workplace attire.

WE BEGIN THE JOURNEY

Who should read this book?

Any woman who is tired of being stuck in an image rut, who dreads getting dressed, who hates her closet, who never knows what to wear, who has trouble finding clothes that flatter her so she abhors shopping, who needs a style revamp, who wants to make a statement with her look but doesn't know where to start, or who desires to take her image into the stratosphere.

In a nutshell, if looking good is important to you, consider this book your style companion. It will take you step by step through everything that impacts your image, from determining your best colors and understanding your shape and proportions to creating a signature style that is authentic to you. And naturally there is tons of advice on getting your wardrobe on track and dressing strategically so you spotlight your assets and minimize your challenge areas.

Oh, and did I mention this book is interactive? It sure is! Like any self-improvement book, you can't just read it passively and put it down and hope that by osmosis you will miraculously experience change. You need to participate by implementing the advice in these pages, completing the short exercises at the end of each chapter and being accountable to your goals. I can tutor you, but ultimately you have to do the work to achieve the results you desire.

Are you ready to start this amazing journey with me?

I promise you that by the end of this book, you will see yourself evolving, and others will start to notice. You will get compliments about how great you look, which will empower you to do even more to boost your image. You will begin to experience getting dressed as an exciting part of your daily rituals because it will become more effortless. You will soon find yourself loving all the clothes in your closet and wanting to show the world how beautiful and fabulous you are!

Take a moment to give yourself permission to hold that bigger, brighter, more fabulous vision of yourself in your mind and know that THAT woman really is you. Just give her the permission to shine.

And to *Flaunt It*, of course.

Chapter One

Dressing with Intention

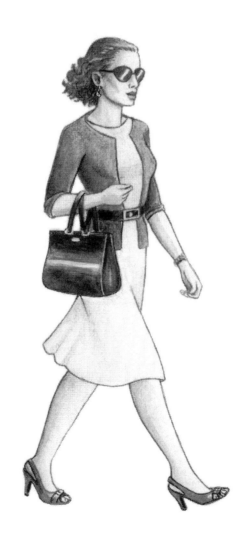

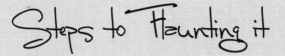

Steps to Flaunting it

- First impressions matter, and you have less than 60 seconds to make that first impression count.

- Image is everything. At first blush, people judge you primarily on the way you look, and you often don't get a second chance.

- Your image must be created with purpose and intent so that the image you convey is WHO you are and HOW you want to be perceived by others.

- Your image must be aligned with your personal goals, lifestyle, personality and preferences for it to be an authentic reflection of you.

- Think of yourself as a brand and you'll dress and act accordingly.

- When you look good, you feel more confident. You are treated with more respect. People are attracted to you, and you have an essence that becomes magnetic.

MAKE YOUR FIRST IMPRESSION A POWERFUL ONE

We've all heard the saying, "You never get a second chance to make a good first impression." If you haven't heard it, guess what? You'd better remember it, because it's true.

In fact, in the first 30 seconds people make at least 12 assumptions about you based on what they see. That's right; you have *less than one minute* to impress someone you just met. Scary thought, huh?

No, not really. Not if you've taken the time, energy and intent to make sure that the image you convey is the image you *want* to convey. That's what this chapter is all about.

So, what things are we judged on in those first precious seconds? Based on appearance alone, people make assumptions about our intelligence, our competency, our educational level, our personality, our achievements, our level of success, our worldliness, our sense of humor, our social heritage, our *savoir faire* and a host of other characteristics.

I'm sure you know exactly what I'm talking about, because we all do it, often unconsciously. Someone walks into a room, and you look her up and down (of course, without her noticing!)—from the color of her lipstick to the freckles on her nose to the style of shoes she's wearing and whether they match her outfit. In an instant, you've determined exactly what kind of woman she is.

Often when I do seminars, I show participants a photo of a woman who is really dressed down (jeans, running shoes, baggy shirt, etc.) and I ask them what they think about her. Time after time I get responses including: she doesn't care how she looks, she's a busy mom, she is doing errands, or some variation of she is not pulled together.

Interestingly, it's not until I point out that it's the same in real life, that we are often judged for better or worse solely on the way we look, then their faces show a deeper awareness of the ways they may be judged. I call the woman "Sally" and I share with them that we just made a bunch of assumptions about Sally based on a photo. And then, I have them imagine 3D Sally—the living breathing version of a woman like her and how their judgments might be even harsher in real life. No one ever disagrees.

In fact, it's not just a vague perception that suggests we are judged on our image first and foremost. In the 1980s, Dr. Albert Mehrabian, a socio linguist, conducted research that found we constantly send "silent messages".

Dr. Mehrabian's research confirmed that 55% of first impressions are based on our visual presentation; 35% are based on vocal cues (the way we communicate, our tone of voice, inflection, etc.); and only 7% are based on what we actually say.

You could be the smartest person in the room, but if your image is at odds with what you are saying, your credibility will be seriously diminished. The bottom line? Your image is talking for you before you even open your mouth!

PRESENCE WITH A PURPOSE ™

Unfortunately, we live in a world where image IS everything. You need to take care of this valuable asset, and yes, it is an asset. If used successfully, your image can position you for the success you desire professionally and personally.

Whether you are vying for a promotion, hoping to impress a new man, an upwardly mobile professional, looking for a new job, a starlet on the make, starting a new business venture, seeking a visible position in your local community, or desiring to be a strong role model for your daughter, your presence needs to be *consistently* polished, pulled together and credible.

'Presence with a Purpose'™ is my tagline, the foundation of my work. Let's talk a bit about what it means.

Start by asking yourself these two questions:

- What image do I project to others?

- How do I want to be perceived?

Your responses to these questions are the building blocks of an image created with *intent*. The dictionary defines intent as: *"purpose; design; meaning or significance."* So in other words, Presence With a Purpose™ conveys that sense of projecting an image that has intention and has meaning, purpose and significance.

Let me explain that a bit more fully.

The package that makes up "you" needs to be aligned with your lifestyle, goals, preferences, personality and core values. You can only project outwardly what you inherently believe to be true about yourself.

Let's have a look at a scenario I'm sure you are familiar with.

You wake up and know deep inside it's going to be a "bad hair day". You take a look in the mirror and think "blahhh!"

After showering, you open the closet and moan before grabbing the beige suit that looks about as drab as you feel. You moan again while getting dressed, and with the same amount of energy required by an Olympic weightlifter, you begrudgingly pull the teal scarf off the rack to add a badly needed touch of color to your sallow cheeks. A touch of lipstick and a dab of blush, and you're out the door.

And wouldn't you know it? Today of all days you are asked to meet the new Marketing Director. There's no time to go home and change. All you can do is pull yourself together as best you can and face the challenge, knowing you don't quite look the part.

In this scenario, did you get dressed with intention? Of course you didn't. You simply slapped on clothes as a functional activity, without passion, thought or motivation, and certainly without intent, purpose or strategy.

We've all been there. But here's the real truth: it is highly likely you're going to feel as "blahhh" for the rest of the day as you did when you got dressed in your "blahhh" mood. Because your outfit, your demeanor and your attitude are all a reflection of how you feel about yourself, unfortunately that is how the rest of the world is going to view you—as "blahhh" or frumpy. That's not what you want now, is it? You really want to be fabulous—whatever that means to you.

Presence With A Purpose™ doesn't mean that you're not going to have "bad hair days". What it means is that on those days, you intensify your commitment to dressing with purpose by asking yourself: What am I trying to achieve today? How do I want to look? What messages do I want to send out? And you dress with those goals in mind.

Let's picture a different scenario.

Imagine you woke up in a "blahhh" mood, but instead of getting dressed according to your mood, you got dressed according to your goals for the day. So let's assume you had an important meeting and your goal was to project confidence and command. You would intentionally select your "power red" peplum jacket that fits you impeccably and pair that with your favorite black pencil skirt. You would accessorize with your wine leather sling back shoes, your white drop pearl earrings and one of your signature watches. You would spend extra time on your hair and makeup to ensure the end result is polished and pulled together. And you'd switch to your croc embossed green tote for just that touch of élan. The result? A look that is completely in synch with your goals for the day.

When you dress with purpose, knowing the colors that make your skin come to life, the correct fit for your shape and the accessories that get you noticed, the overall vibe you give off is magnetic. And that is powerful.

ARE YOU A CHRISTIAN LOUBOUTIN OR A JIMMY CHOO?

We each have a personal brand (a persona) we express to others, through the way we look, dress, behave and communicate. Your goal is to ensure that your image maximizes your brand and sends out the right messages about you.

A company's brand has to do with its reputation, how it is perceived in the marketplace and how much cache its logo carries. In the same way, each of us is our own walking advertisement—our own personal brand. Get the picture?

Think of Nike's "Just Do It!" marketing campaign and what it did for the Nike brand. Or better yet, De Beer's famous "A Diamond Is Forever" campaign that began way back in the 1940s. Now that's a slogan most women can relate to!

Our personal brand conveys information about our credibility, intelligence, self-image, confidence and so much more. All these factors impact our reputation in the eyes of others.

So ask yourself: What does your "brand" say about you? Would you be more attuned to it if it was YOU in the Nordstrom's store window display?

If you think of your external image as your "packaging" and your internal self-image as your "product offering", then they have to be aligned or the end result is not authentic. After all, how would you feel if you opened the elegant Tiffany & Co gift box you've just been given to discover a rhinestone inside?

Every woman has a unique life situation, personality and purpose, which impacts how she will be perceived and how she perceives herself. Just as Christian Louboutin pumps are differentiated from other designer shoes by their signature red soles, and Cole Haan shoes are designed with Nike Air technology, so we each have our own unique image "package." What is yours? Your personal brand hinges on establishing a reputation for yourself, showcasing what differentiates you from other women and conveying these qualities in every situation and encounter. It says: this woman has her act together!

Developing a strong personal brand takes effort, focus and deep soul searching. Play to your strengths—those qualities that come naturally to you. Start by building a strong foundation for your personal brand built on the qualities of authenticity, credibility, expertise and reputation.

FROM FRUMPY TO FABULOUS

When you look good and are dressed in ways that flatter you, the benefits can be enormous. You feel confident and self-assured. You get constant validation from those who compliment you because you look amazing. People are automatically attracted to you. You have an extra edge to use to your advantage. You have "presence" and get noticed. You just *feel* good knowing you look good. Why wouldn't any woman want these benefits?

Come on, be honest. If you had no limitation, no boundaries and the sky was the limit, wouldn't you want to be fabulous? Better yet, wouldn't you love the power that comes with the ability to Flaunt It?

To conclude, let's finish with a short exercise. And no, this is NOT an exam and you WON'T get graded! The exercises at the end of each chapter are simply a way for you to get the most value out of this book and to begin the process of transforming yourself from frumpy to fabulous. After all, if you absorb all this great information and advice I'm sharing with you and diligently do the exercises at the end of each chapter, you won't recognize yourself by the end of this book! You'll come to see that the art of dressing well and looking great can be effortless once you evolve into your very own personal style expert. And ladies, when you are reveling in your magnificence, you absolutely will be Flaunting It.

BECOMING FABULOUS

Make a list of positive words that you want people to associate with you. In other words, think very deeply about what you want your image to project when others see you. What do you want them to think? Perhaps you want to be seen as one or more of the following: wealthy, warm, attractive, confident, fun, unconventional, serious, soft, competent, happy, one of a kind, strong, approachable, successful, etc.

Go for it! Those were just a few ideas to get you going. Start writing down as many adjectives that come to mind at first then go back and edit the list so you have 7 unique words that really resonate for you. These "descriptors" will become the start of your new image created with purpose and intent. You can create separate lists for your personal and professional life.

If you are unsure about which words to choose, ask a family member, colleague or friend to describe you. If you are not happy with their choice of descriptions, now is the time to decide for yourself how you can change/upscale your image so others see you more favorably.

Throughout the course of this book, you will be working with these "key words", as they will help you define your unique personal style and create a purposeful and powerful presence.

Chapter Two

Getting Creative with Color

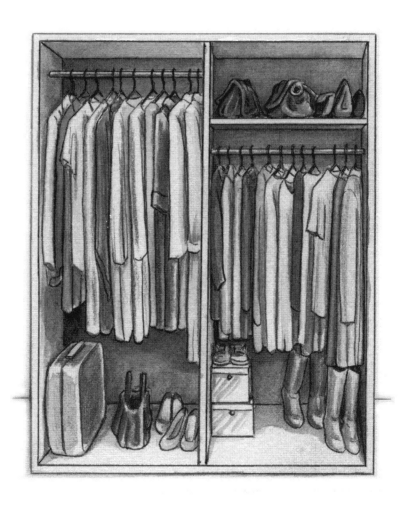

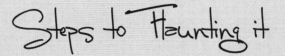

Steps to Flaunting it

✔ Color is your best friend, so learn how to use it to your advantage by wearing your "power colors" to add impact to your image.

✔ Experiment with color until you find the ones that make you "zing" with life and vitality. Choose those that make you look vibrant, younger and more beautiful.

✔ Different shades have different characteristics, so add impact to the image you want to convey by wearing them strategically. For example, wear red to convey confidence, blue to convey reliability, pink to convey femininity or fuchsia to convey pizzazz.

✔ Be bold! Once you've discovered your unique palette, wear it with confidence. If you prefer, add splashes of your colors by accessorizing with scarves, jewelry, belts, bags and shoes.

✔ Have fun mixing and matching colors to express your style and creativity.

Color is your most powerful friend in the wardrobe. It can transform you from drab to fab with the flick of a fuchsia fingernail or the swish of a scarlet scarf, as long as the colors you wear are in the right tones and hues for you.

Embracing your personal color palette is so transformative. It energizes your wardrobe, boosts and enhances your appearance, and adds creative flair to your image.

One of the first questions I get asked by new clients is: "But how do I know which colors work for me?"

That's what we're going to discuss now—the strategic use of flattering colors that work with your natural tones to raise you above the sea of familiar beige, black, navy and gray, so you can grab that "wow" factor and shake it for all it's worth.

The important thing to remember before we go any further is that it doesn't cost any more to establish a color presence. That putty blouse on the rack is likely to cost just the same as the peacock blue one that could boost your appearance into the stratosphere.

Think about your favorite color right now. Let's imagine it is green. If you like green that much you probably have quite a few shades in your closet, some that look great on you and some that fall flat. I have a client, Dana, who loves green. She had emerald, mint, forest, lime, olive and sage shades in her closet. But lime green looks truly awful on her, and forest is a bit too somber and makes the dark circles under her eyes more apparent. Olive washes her out and makes her look drab. Sage green is nice and soft but it does not have the "wow" factor for her. But emerald! Emerald looks stunning on her. Her skin looks radiant, the green in her eyes sparkle that much more and her hair looks more luminous. Emerald is a power color for Dana. Mint is quirky and fun and is a tone she can wear as an accent or when she wants to convey a more playful energy.

This is just one example of a few shades of *one* color. I'm trying to reinforce the point that the choice of colors you can wear is virtually endless and therefore can be overwhelming to you. You may stick to wearing the same "safe" color palette all the time because you have too many options to choose from and are scared to make the wrong choices.

I hope after reading this chapter you are set free and are eager to explore all the yummy colors waiting for you. Every woman has a unique palette that can truly transform her looks. You just have to know your "wow" colors.

So let's start first with the basics.

ARE YOU WARM OR COOL?

Everybody's skin has either warm or cool tones or somewhere in between, no matter what their ethnicity.

To start with the basics, let's go back to grade school painting classes. Remember how there are 3 primary colors: yellow, red and blue? Well, that's where we're going to start so you can work out which skin type you are, if you don't already know.

Using red as the base color, by adding yellow to it you eventually end up with orange. Anywhere along that color wheel from yellow to red are the warm colors, so if your skin has golden tones, or is true beige in complexion, then you are considered warm.

If you start with red and move towards the blue end of the color wheel, the hues along that side are considered to be cool tones. So if your skin has bluish undertones, or your skin is alabaster white, you can be considered cool.

Skin tone and eye color are the primary indicators of your color category and to a lesser extent hair color. It is the skin, eye and hair combo that gives each person their unique color stamp. Got it?

Indicators for the woman whose colors are on the warm end of the spectrum:

- If she is a natural red head or has freckles, she is hands down warm.

- She has reddish tones in her hair, or is strawberry blonde, or has a very rich warm brown hair color.

- Her skin is golden brown, beige or peachy.

- When she greys, her hair will have a yellowish tinge so it will need to be dyed.

- Eyes are hazel, medium to light brown, soft blue or green.

- Colors like khaki or grey can wash her out.

- Great colors are rich browns, emerald green, rusts, cranberry, tomato red, teal blue, bubble gum pink.

Indicators for the woman whose colors are on the cool end of the spectrum:

- Skin is alabaster white or porcelain or has pink undertones.

- Eyes are very dark—black or dark brown—or jewel toned.

- When hair greys, it goes silvery with no hint of yellow.

- True strong colors tend to be the most flattering: black, rich purple, cobalt blue, forest green, fuchsia. Icy pastels can also look great on her.

- Colors like brown, rust, and orange look awful on her.

If you cross between these two categories, you're likely, a mix of warm and cool.

WELL-KNOWN CELEBRITIES AND THEIR COLOR TONES

Taking a peek at some well-known celebrities and their color palette may also help you decide whereabouts on the color spectrum you fall.

Blonde beauties like Gwyneth Paltrow and Nicole Kidman with their milky-white skin and ice blue eyes should tell you they are both "cool" customers. The porcelain skin and dark hair and eyes of Anne Hathaway and Jennifer Connelly also place them at the cooler end of the spectrum. Black beauties like Iman and Naomi Campbell are also on the cool color spectrum.

Sultry blondes like Kate Hudson with her hazel-green eyes and Drew Barrymore with her beige skin and brown eyes (and hair that goes from blonde to red depending on her mood!) make them true "warm" personalities. So do skin tones like the golden glow of Beyonce or Jennifer Lopez, both warm. Generally most natural red heads like Julianne Moore are warm as well.

While dark haired beauties like Catherine Zeta-Jones "zing" in cool shades like magenta, they also look fabulous in warmer tones, or simple black and white, making them more of a mix on the color spectrum. The same goes for a stunner like Halle Berry. But, don't misunderstand; if you are a mix of both warm and cool tones you are lucky enough to look fabulous in colors from both sides of the color wheel. So your chances of messing up your colors are that much slimmer.

HAVING FUN WITH COLOR

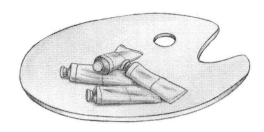

While we're on the topic of grade school painting classes, do you remember how much fun it was when you got to put on your little apron, grab hold of a huge paint brush and a virtual rainbow of paints and color to your heart's content?

I'll bet painting class rarely saw any sad faces, tantrums or tears. It was a time for expressing yourself, for your imagination to run wild and your little fingers to capture whatever you were feeling on paper. Who cared if mommy was painted purple and daddy was green? The sun was generally bright, shiny yellow and the chimney red, or did you see things differently? It didn't really matter—it was all about the beauty of the colors and how happy they made you feel.

Wouldn't it be wonderful if you could recapture those vivid moments of innocent creativity now with your wardrobe?

Well, I'm going to let you in on a little secret; you can! Your wardrobe can express all that imagination and creativity you had when you were a child with the inventive use of colors that ignite your image and express your essence. And all it takes is the know-how to understand which colors add the ka-pow factor and which colors go ka-plop.

The general rule of thumb is easy: if you are warm toned, choose colors from the warm end of the spectrum or alternatively warm hues of cool colors (for example a teal blue versus a royal blue). If you are cool toned, choose colors from the cool end of the spectrum, or alternatively cool tones of warm colors (for example jade green versus hunter). If you are a mix of warm and cool, you have a wider color palette to choose from (you lucky gal!), and you can choose according to what suits you and makes you go "zing".

Another great rule of thumb is that you can generally always wear the same color as your eyes and make an impact. Try it and you'll see what I mean.

An important point! The true impact of color is seen by the colors we wear from the waist up. So we need to get the right tones in shirts, blouses, jackets, camis, Tees, dresses and any accessories like scarves and jewelry. Remember, color is determined by our skin, eyes and hair so it's the colors we wear closest to our face that make us stun or snooze.

Regarding the colors of your pants and skirts, you just want to be sure you match the colors you wear on the bottom with the ones on the top, so your entire ensemble works for you. For instance, if you love tan but it looks awful near your face, you can certainly wear it in a skirt or slacks, if you pair it with a complementary color on top that looks amazing.

Contrary to popular myth, most women can wear most colors, (with the exception of yellows and purples, the extremes of warm and cool respectively) depending on the hue, tone, tint or shade of that color. Choosing the right tone can turn you from blah to zing in seconds, (or as long as it takes to hold a piece of fabric against your skin).

When I'm introducing a new client to the wide world of colors and the immediate impact they can have, I like to start with various shades of red. Red is a strong, dynamic color with a multitude of tonal variations and a really strong color personality, so it's easy to see which tones look great and which tones fall flat against a woman's face. Besides, red is the most versatile of all the primary colors and works well with almost any neutral you have in your wardrobe. I also like to try to find, what I call, a woman's "super hero red"—the red that makes her look emboldened, strong, confident and powerful—like she could command a troop if she wanted. Really wearing this shade of red is like a secret weapon that you can use to charm a man or chair a meeting. Aren't you really curious now to find out?

I believe every woman can wear a shade in the red family, from the warmest coral red to the bluest raspberry hue. You may have to trust me on this.

You can try this exercise at home, but it's better to head to a department store where there are a wide variety of colors to choose from, many you may not have thought to experiment with in the past. Try to do this in natural lighting if possible for the most accurate result. And take your gal pal with you. After all, what are we without our girlfriends for support and advice?

I like to start with what I call the "happy" reds. These are the reds with slight tones of yellow in them, so they are vibrant, bright and warm because they lean towards the orange end of the scale. Pick a top in that shade off the rack and hold it up, close to your face. How does it make you look?

With red, you'll know instantly whether you are working it or it is working you. And when you find your super hero red, you'll notice the strength, confidence and command it imbues you with.

Generally, when colors work for you, your face looks energized and glowing; you look radiant, your eyes sparkle and you'll "pop". If the color works against you, it will make you look washed out or ashen, your eyes won't look as bright, you may notice dark circles under your eyes, your natural color will disappear or you'll look overwhelmed. Do you see why it's so important to nail your best colors?

Keep going with our experiment here. Move on to a red with less yellow—a "poppy red"—and look at yourself in the mirror once again. How does a less yellowy red make you look?

Surprisingly, many women who thought they could never wear red wear poppy red beautifully. It is a warm, radiant hue that is a "wow" color for many women. However, it may not be one of your signature colors; if so, move on to a richer shade of tomato red.

Tomato red is a virtual true red, with almost no yellow or blue tones to influence it. Don't be concerned if it seems too strong for your coloring. A true tomato red is very intense and can be overwhelming on a lot of women. It's simply the mid way point in the range of reds.

Next, move on to a claret colored top. We are now moving in to the cooler tones, so if you find yourself saying "yuk" instantly, you know you are definitely a true warm tone.

While claret may or may not be one of your signature colors, move on to the next color in the scale, a deeper maroon, and try it up against your face. Once again, it will either sing or suck.

By now, you should have determined which of the reds make you bloom with life—your "super hero red". When you wear this shade, you can stop traffic. Seriously! No doubt, you'll have driven the shop assistant (and your girlfriend) crazy, so you can happily conclude today's exercise. Did you have fun?

The most delightful thing I find when doing this exercise with clients using my color drapes, with the full spectrum of greens, blues, orange/peach, pink/salmon, purple, yellow and reds, is how often they say, "I never realized I could wear this color!" And they get such a kick out of discovering a brand new shade they can confidently add to their wardrobe because they've seen for themselves how much snap, crackle and pop that color gives them. Let's take a look at a color analysis success story.

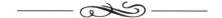

TRANSFORMATION IN ACTION
MEET LOUANN

Louann is an ebony complexioned, attractive black woman. And boy, did she love the color beige. She wore head to toe beige routinely. It was her absolute favorite color. The trouble was, beige on Louann looked just awful! It blended right into her beige colored skin, brown hair and eyes, and fell completely flat. All variations of beige/tan/ taupe were an absolute snooze on her. As I conducted her color analysis, Louann was amazed at how radiant she looked in colors she would never ever wear like peach, coral, sunburst yellow, tangerine, and others. And sure enough, mid way through our session, she reached the undoubtable conclusion—she needed to stop wearing beige! It was a watershed moment for her; a color she adored because she associated it with sand, and all the fond memories she shared going to the beach every weekend with her family. But all was not lost. I assured Louann she could surround herself in beige with accessories, and in her home. And of course she could wear beige pants and skirts till the cows came home!

Observation: Our color associations can run deep. I have seen similar patterns time and time again with women. Pay attention to what people say when you wear certain colors. You want to hear, "that color looks great on you" or "you look beautiful in that dress" and not, "I love that color top". The latter compliment does not necessarily mean the color is right for you. In Louann's case many of her friends had been begging her to stop wearing beige. But she couldn't see what they saw until she saw that color in relation to the full spectrum of colors. Her emotional association with the color beige was so strong because it went all the way back to her childhood. If everyone is telling you that a particular color does not suit you, listen. Chances are they're right. You can adore a color but it doesn't mean you need to wear it if it does nothing for you.

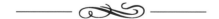

The trick is to continue this exercise with all the primary colors so you can discover all the wonderful tones and hues that transform your style from dull to wow in an instant. But the sure fire way to know your signature colors is to have them done profession-ally, especially if your girlfriend happens to be color blind. You can find an image consultant who will use a variety of techniques, including draping you with different fabrics, to help you discover your optimal colors.

Often when clients have their colors professionally done, they eventually recognize the colors that add the "wow" factor to their image; their eyes start to become trained to see the nuances of a warm blue versus a cool blue or a soft blue versus a vivid blue and they begin to truly *see* which of those tones is most enhancing for them and why.

PLAYING STRATEGICALLY IN THE COLOR SANDBOX

"We are what we wear." How's that for a cutting-edge new slogan? But it's true.

As we discussed in Chapter 1, our image and the way we present ourselves tell people a surprising amount about us in a very short space of time. And we didn't even get to mention color in that chapter.

The power colors we choose to wear—those that intensify our strengths—not only identify us as individuals, but they can leave an indelible mark on those we interact with.

Learn to make color your fashion ally, and be bold. When you catch a glimpse of yourself in the mirror in one of your power colors, that image smiling back at you has the ability to magically transform you. Seeing the brighter, more confident, more self-assured person in the mirror instantly creates those positive attributes inside, so you shine inwardly as well as outwardly.

Every primary, secondary and tertiary color is associated with unique core attributes which can be conveyed to the wearer of that color. For example, if you wore your "super hero red", the attributes we associate with strong red, like assertiveness, confidence, authority, allure and passion, will translate to you too. Isn't that exciting? In this way you can begin to use color strategically. Want to attract that charming man you've had your eyes on? Wear a killer dress in your "super hero" red.

There are countless colors to choose from to use strategically. Add a dribble of white to red and you get pink, which has an entirely new and unique set of characteristics. Pink is soft and feminine in its purest form, demure, understated yet romantic. Some women look best in pinks.

Add a dash of blue to pink and you get fuchsia, with an altogether new set of attributes. Fuchsia is bold, sassy, dramatic and exciting.

Similarly, turquoise is a shade of blue that is warmer in tone but it can have more "zing" than a navy blue. Blue as a whole is seen as trustworthy and safe. Turquoise, though, says fun, free-spirited and engaging. Navy, on the other hand, is serious and authoritative. Both blues, but both send different vibes.

Do you wish to look upbeat and cheerful? Wear yellow or orange. Do you need to be more approachable? Green is your friend. Regal and elegant? Purple is your hue.

Do you see where I'm going with this?

Every color and every hue within it has its own unique characteristics that you too can embrace. You have a variety of colors to choose from. Start using them strategically so you can create your desired impact.

The best piece of advice I can offer is to explore the colors you love most and then work out which tones within those colors make you "pop" and come to life. These colors become your "power colors" and best friends; and like any friends, you'll want to find out as much about them as you possibly can. The Internet has plenty of information about the psychology of colors. Learn how your favorite colors can infuse you with attributes to help you look your best and further your intent for each occasion.

Additionally, look to nature for inspiration. Observe the brilliant color palette of a South American Macau or the magnificent displays of color in tropical plants like Bird of Paradise to help you see the playful interaction of colors upon colors.

WOWING WITH COLOR

A question I'm often asked is which colors go with each other. While there are a few basic rules of thumb I will share here, I want to encourage you to follow your own instincts. I've found women are often scared to make a mistake, so they play it very safe with color, sticking to neutrals like black, navy, brown or beige and ignoring all the vibrant, soft, energetic, or fun tones that non-neutrals can provide. Color is meant to be enjoyed and can reinforce your personal style and pull together your image. Use this free asset!

So let's tackle **RULE #1**: Neutrals can virtually be worn with any other color, and **RULE #2**: Any neutral can be paired with another neutral. Yes! So stop agonizing about what colored pants to wear with your favorite teal blouse.

In case you are wondering, the core neutrals are black, white, grey, brown, and navy. So let's explore how we can get creative with our color pairings using neutrals as a foundation.

White is clean and fresh. It brightens up other colors it is paired with. In the summer, a pair of white slacks can be paired with any colored top or print and look amazing. I am partial to white bottoms in the warmer months because white makes colors pop so we see their true essence. Bright colors such as yellow, orange or turquoise look more vibrant when paired with white.

Black on the other hand, while the default neutral for many women, can sometimes overpower other colors it's paired with. Imagine a fuchsia top with a white skirt then imagine the same top with black slacks. Do you visualize the difference? One is not 'better' than the other, but I do want you to understand these subtle nuances. If you want to downplay a bright color, pair it with a dark neutral. But if you want it enlivened, pair it with white.

Black: The fastest path to effortless. A woman's closet would have a huge gap without a basic black skirt and black dress slacks. Black bottoms are very versatile and so effortless when paired with other items. Black is perhaps the ultimate neutral. It also helps that it is the most slimming of colors for women who want to contain their curves. Any color, (seriously *ANY* color) works with black. If you are not confident about color matching, black is your friend. Pair it with color, neutrals or prints. It works with them all.

Then there is grey. **Grey** is safe and predictable but it is one of those mid-tone neutrals that looks great because it does not compete as much with the colors it's paired with. A grey suit is an excellent choice for many women, rather than black, which on fair, soft features can often be too stark. Grey and pink are a natural combination and look amazing paired together on top (as in grey blazer, pink blouse). Grey and red is an unusual combination, but one that works. Grey and white is crisp, clean and sharp.

Brown is earthy and warm and comes in a variety of tones from tan and beige to chocolate. Brown is typically seen as boring, but it can be a very rich neutral if paired with the right colors. If brown is a good color on you, it can make you look inviting and approachable. I love brown and wear it often as a rich neutral. Brown coupled with a soft blue is a natural combination. I also love brown and ivory or brown and red. On me, the latter is a slamming combo. Medium-light brown (such as a tan) can work with a hot color like orange to tone it down a little.

Navy is a business staple. And no wonder, as it is perceived as trustworthy, stable and professional. Navy and white are both neutrals, and just like the sea which inspired this combo, it is a fresh, crisp and clean pairing. Navy also looks great with lighter shades of blue like turquoise or powder blue. Pink softens the starkness of a navy jacket and so makes for a great combination. Navy and red, on the other hand, is a strong and powerful pairing.

So now that you know how to use neutrals in more creative ways with other colors, let us explore some other creative color pairings, so you will be inspired to try a few of your own. But first, a few more "rules".

RULE #3: Colors at opposite ends of the color wheel make very dramatic pairings. **RULE #4:** Hues closer to each other on the color wheel create easy complements to each other, which convey a softer effect. **RULE #5:** To create an interesting monochromatic look, use varying shades of the same color in your outfit. For example, an ensemble of mint, sage and lime green, will be a more creative way to rock a monochromatic look compared to wearing mint green from top to bottom.

Let's look at some more creative color pairings.

Many women shy away from wearing pure **yellow,** and rightly so, as it can be tricky to wear well. Darker skinned, tanned and olive complexions most compliment this hue. Buttercup yellow looks amazing with burnt orange, bright red and rust. I also like this hue with gecko green. Imagine a burnt orange dress paired with a buttercup yellow cardigan or a yellow Tee with red shorts. See how fun this can be?

Emerald **green** looks wonderful with a light orange or melon hue. Olive green looks smashing with mustard. Forest green can be paired with sea foam green (a blue/green) for instant oomph factor.

Turquoise is a great hue for spring and summer. I love a turquoise top with a yellow skirt. Very fun. Turquoise and white is also a pretty pairing, as is turquoise and pale green. Turquoise and fuchsia is a very dramatic look. Pale soft blue works to soften harsher colors like navy, burgundy, or black. It's also very striking with almost any mid-tone green or sea foam green. Just avoid pairing turquoise or light blues with black —the black sobers these colors up way too much.

Royal purple is so intense and powerful. The trick to wearing this color is using it as your base and adding other complements to make it soar. Purple and yellow are opposites on the color wheel but are a great pairing for the woman who can handle strong contrast in her colors. For a subtler effect, try rich purple with olive or with salmon. Violet and fuchsia can be a sassy combo.

Red is actually a fabulous accent color as well as a primary one. Some people count red as a neutral as it goes beautifully with so many colors. Tomato red, pink and white are a very feminine combo. Raspberry red and orange are very creative together. And coral with burgundy is a nice subtle pairing. Wine red and teal can be stunning. And of course there is the power pairing, red and black, standard in so many suit ensembles.

Orange, my favorite color, is best when toned down a notch. I love pairing orange with rust and brown for a very earthy combination. Orange also looks striking with cranberry red. For a lighter vibe try apricot (light orange) with a blush toned pink. For real drama, pair orange with mid-tone blue—opposites on the color wheel.

Pink is a very forgiving color on many women, but some shy away from it because it is seen as so girlie. Not so! Pink can be sexy and spicy especially in its richer hues. Fuchsia is a definite favorite on my list and paired with earthy brown is a crowd pleaser. I love the femininity of pure pink and white—very Lilly Pulitzer. Speaking of which, the designer often pairs bubble gum pink with a soft green like mint, another excellent combo. Warm deep pink is great with turquoise. And soft blush with tan or beige makes for a lovely neutral monochromatic palette.

Phew!! And we've only scratched the surface here. The point is, the options for expressing your creativity and personality using color are endless. When you start incorporating three and four color combos into your ensembles it gets really interesting. What I've tried to do in this section is inspire and encourage you to experiment, play and have fun mixing and matching colors.

Playing with Color: The fastest path to effortless. Wear your best colors in combinations that look smashing on you.

COLOR WITH A PURPOSE

If you're anything like me, after reading that last section your mind must be whirring around with ideas of ways to combine the colors in your closet in new and more creative ways. If you're exactly like me, you'd have taken a break from reading to try out some of these new exciting combos and would have made a list of new colors you *must* have in your closet now. All good stuff!

We're almost done. Let's have a final look at the impact of color on your appearance and examine other ways to optimize your image using colors strategically to add that "ka-pow" factor:

- ❖ The colors you wear from the waist up are the ones that matter, so make them count. They are the colors that enhance or detract from your facial skin tone, eyes and hair, which determine whether you look sensational or not.

- ❖ Wearing colors that complement your skin tone close to your face makes you look and feel healthier, so you look more radiantly beautiful. In fact, your power colors can help smooth out your skin tone, reduce the appearance of dark circles under your eyes and even make expression lines less noticeable, so you look younger.

- ❖ Even though it's the colors waist up that matter the most, be sure to coordinate the colors in your ensemble from top to bottom for optimal impact. So theoretically, if cranberry is an awful shade on you, you can wear it in a skirt and pair it with one of your "wow" colors. Just be sure you match that cranberry bottom with a shade that complements it and more importantly you.

- ❖ Color is more than just looking great; it's about feeling great as well. Certain colors are invigorating and refreshing and enhance our mood when we wear them, while others may pull our mood down and make us feel dour and miserable. It all depends on the wearer, so always wear the hues that invigorate and enliven you.

- ❖ Non-neutral colors tend to make you feel happier, prettier, more upbeat and more feminine. You can also use these shades to dramatically accessorize a neutral wardrobe. If you are a basic black gal, or prefer the neutral shades of grey, tan, navy or beige, use refreshing flashes of color from your palette as accents in tops, scarves, jewelry, bags and shoes.

- ❖ The closer these accents are to your face, the more impact they will have in "lifting" the neutral colors. You can instantly turn your image around with a gorgeous pink silk scarf tied around your neck. Or perhaps you would prefer a brightly colored turquoise necklace or an amazing pair of emerald earrings? Experiment to see what different colors look like against your skin. Be daring and brave.

❖ Make sure YOU wear the color and the color doesn't wear you. A compliment that tells you that you've got it right is: "You look fantastic/beautiful/pretty in that color", and not, "I love that color dress you're wearing".

❖ Many women limit themselves by thinking they can only wear certain colors in specific seasons. They think, "I have to wait for fall to wear that lovely rust hue" or "I can only wear yellow in summer" or some variation of these thoughts. Nonsense. Wear your best colors year round. There are no rules about what time of the year you should wear colors (as in no white after Labor Day—really!). So have fun and enjoy your 'wow' colors throughout the year!

I'd like to close this chapter by relating a story that's absolutely true about the impact your power colors can have on your presence.

I was invited to a five hour business conference that I reluctantly attended. To give myself a much needed energy boost, I selected a conservative dress in tomato red, my "super hero" red.

The conference was being held in Washington DC, which is the veritable home of power black, so as I made my entrance, I was confronted with a sea of black, with a few pops of other neutral shades.

As I made my way through the crowd, I noticed that people everywhere were stopping to look at me. Well, I am used to that. I'm tall (6' 1") so that alone gives me a certain presence. And because I'm an image consultant, who actively practices what she preaches, I'm used to attention. But this situation was ridiculous.

Groups of people seemed to be trying to get my attention wherever I moved, and a couple of men in particular made an effort to introduce themselves to me. I took it all in stride but truly it was a bit much.

In all honesty, I hadn't really given a thought to the effect my red dress would have on this occasion, but my presence was certainly making an impact. It was as if every person in that room wanted to get to know me. I was magnetic.

One particularly handsome gentleman apparently was tailing me all morning, and only minutes before the event concluded, he plucked up the courage to introduce himself to me. His actual words were: "Boy you sure are wearing that red dress." Now, really, what woman doesn't want to hear that compliment! We exchanged business cards and needless to say, ended up dating for 6 months. We are still very good friends today.

The point of the story? Wearing your power colors is powerful! It can impact your ability to achieve success in your endeavors, whether they are personal, professional or both.

BECOMING FABULOUS

First up, determine whether you are warm, cool or a mix of both and then experiment with a variety of colors right across the color spectrum to determine which colors make you pop. Continue with the color draping exercise I recommended during this chapter, and move onto other colors after you've covered red. Examine the hues that make you literally glow and then use those colors to add impact to your wardrobe.

Research, using the Internet and books, to learn the psychological characteristics of your colors so you can use them strategically to add impact to your image.

Be open, bold and have fun!

Chapter Three

Real Women Have Curves

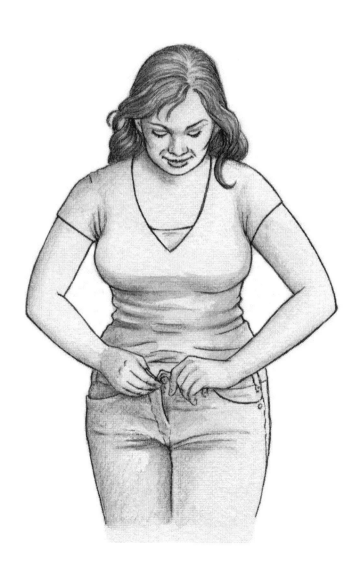

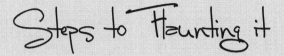

Steps to Flaunting it

✔ Embrace the woman you are. The art of figure flattery is all about enhancing your body's assets and disguising those parts that need a little help.

✔ By understanding which of the 6 basic body shapes you are, you can work towards picking clothing that flatters you and makes you look and feel fabulous.

✔ Eyes up: The fastest path to effortless. When you draw people's eyes up to your neck and face, they cannot help but focus there. Any figure flaws below often go unnoticed because you are working to get their attention up to your face. Hair, makeup, accessories like jewelry and scarves, wearing the right colors and wearing enhancing necklines, all help reinforce "eyes up".

✔ A key to working your look is understanding your proportions and combining that with figure flattery, so you can dress in a way that wows.

✔ There are many strategies to looking taller and slimmer once you understand your body particulars. Use the tips I share here to present a more poised and svelte look.

USE COMPLEMENTS TO GET COMPLIMENTS

Dressing to flatter your figure isn't about hiding your flaws in as much as it's about enhancing your assets. What are your best assets? Is it your strong shoulders? Toned arms? Great shapely legs? Tiny waist? Alluring cleavage? Smooth, well defined back? Nice tush? Rosy, flawless complexion?

Come on, take a moment and do a mental scan - there must be something you absolutely love about you? What have people complimented you on in the past? What do you like about yourself?

This chapter is a celebration of the positives about your body and a lesson on how to play up your assets so you look and feel amazing. I will talk about the main figure types and give you tips on ways to Flaunt and highlight the best about your figure. I will also share tricks to detract attention from the parts you may not love quite as much.

Instead of fighting with your body, work with it. When I work with a woman, I look for the beauty in her—those positive attributes that help her shine—and I work with her to accentuate that beauty.

Highlighting your assets is a wonderful way for people to notice how fabulous you are. Even better, you'll feel so great when you have mastered the art of figure flattery that you'll start to strut your stuff and people will take notice... "Who IS that girl?" You, my friend! So, are you ready to rock 'n roll?

LEARN TO LOVE THE SKIN YOU'RE IN

What is it about women and their bodies? Why is it so challenging for many of us to embrace the body we have *right now* regardless of our age, size or life stage?

As women, we can be so hard on ourselves, and too darn unforgiving. A man will look at his reflection and see the positives. He'll think, "Yeah, this gut is getting smaller everyday." But a woman? She'll see her reflection and angst about her arms, legs, nose, breasts, butt—anything and everything!

And while we're on the subject, did you know that studies have shown we get to see our reflection up to 55 times every day in elevator doors, windows, mirrors, store fronts, bathrooms, and so on. That's a whole lot of times trying to avoid your reflection, or feeling bad about your self every time you do.

Which explains why some women suddenly find themselves in an image rut. They stopped paying attention, didn't take care of their assets or ceased managing the areas that needed work. They start to hide under their clothes.

Or equally as sad, many women don't give themselves permission to try new styles, colors or designs; so they end up with a wardrobe that bores them or one that doesn't bare the slightest resemblance to the woman they desire to be. The result? They dread getting dressed each day as they have no idea what to wear because what they have in their closet no longer suits them.

Then a day comes when they are caught off guard and do catch their reflection in the mirror, or see a recent photo of themselves and they are shocked. What happened to me, they wonder?

What happened to her? She stopped caring or stopped allowing herself to be inspired to look great. She no longer made her image a priority in her life. It became an after thought or no thought at all. Life took over and at some point, she lost the essence of who she was. Her clothing reflected her lack of interest. Perhaps she bought clothing for comfort. Or she grabbed things in the store for one function or the other because she needed something to wear and shopped under duress. Perhaps she started to just stick with what worked, and wore the same type of ensembles over and over. Perhaps, she never even really knew what to look for in clothing to make her look fabulous.

How can you Flaunt what you don't even know you have?

Am I talking to you? I'm here to assure you it is okay. I've witnessed how getting stuck in an image rut slowly creeps in until wham! You're in one. The good news is you can get out of your rut and start the transformation to a more fabulous you, right now. This is precisely why you are reading this book—to get the help and advice you need so you end up knowing the clothing that suits you, loving your wardrobe and excited to get dressed each and every day.

My own testimonial? In my late teens, I had a poor self-image. I didn't like the way I looked. I felt (*get this?*) too skinny, too gawky and unattractive. And hard as it may be to believe when you're over 6', I wanted to be invisible. Invisible!

Now, many years older and wiser, when I look at old photos of myself I see a beautiful young woman. Gorgeous even. How could I not see that then? All I know is that I didn't.

When I had my "aha" moment over 15 years ago, I made a pact with myself. I promised I would always be at peace with my appearance; that I would see the beauty in me; and that I would embrace my stellar stature. No more invisible Natalie.

Now when I look at my reflection, I see many parts of my body I absolutely love; and yes, I see parts that if I had a magic wand I would probably change. But I don't dwell much on those, especially if, short of magic, there is nothing I could do to change them. I focus on what I can enhance, highlight and Flaunt: my killer smile, my long legs, my strong shoulders, my beautiful hands, my gracefully long neck, my tiny waist and my cute perky bustline. And I've learned to embrace those less than ideal aspects too, because they are part of the whole that makes me "me".

I urge you to practice this too. You need to be as loving to yourself and your body as you would like others to be toward you. And it starts with you. It's you who needs to have the positive self-image first. No one can give it to you; it has to be a gift you give to yourself.

Start right now and do something amazing for yourself that can transform your life. Give yourself the gift of self-love.

UNDERSTANDING YOUR BODY'S UNIQUE BEAUTY & SHAPE

No one's body is exactly like yours. Your body is as unique as you are. That's why understanding how to dress your body will help you create a figure flattering image every time you get dressed.

Body typing is essentially looking at how your shoulders relate to your hips and assessing whether or not you have a defined waist. When the hips and shoulders are the same width and there is a defined waist, the figure is considered balanced. Once you become acquainted with your own particular shape and discover what to enhance, what to minimize, where you are wide, where you are narrow and the tactics you can use to appear taller, slimmer and more balanced, you will look and feel so much better in your clothes. It is really that simple.

Speaking of simple, let's review a few basic rules.

RULE #1: you want to visually widen where you are narrow and visually narrow where you are wide. **RULE #2:** Vertical lines or design elements elongate and slim. That is because they draw the eyes up and down. Horizontal lines or design elements widen and shorten, because they draw the eyes from side to side. **RULE #3:** Diagonal lines or design elements force the eyes to move across the body so they are great for detracting and camouflaging wide or bulgy areas of the body. The same is true of patterns. **RULE #4: Fastest path to effortless:** Employ the "eyes up" technique. Use accessories, including jewelry, scarves, pins; your power colors in tops, jackets, dresses and accessories; interesting and figure flattering necklines; your hair and makeup; etc., to draw the eye of the onlooker constantly back to your face. The point is, if you keep their eyes focused on your face, they won't be paying attention to the fact that you may be a bit hippy or that your thighs might be on the larger side—they'll be too fixated on your face and all the eyes up tactics you're using to notice. This really works as a detractor technique. Trust me.

In the sections following, we'll examine the essential features of the 6 basic body shapes: Ideal, Triangle, Inverted Triangle, Hourglass, Round and Rectangle. For each figure, we'll look at the most flattering pants, dress and top to suit that figure type, so you'll know exactly the types of designs, cuts and accents to select to look great.

You will be armed with tons of advice and information to help you master dressing your body to flatter your figure effectively. And guess what? After combining this new knowledge with your color mastery from the prior chapter, you'll be nearly halfway on the road to looking fabulous!

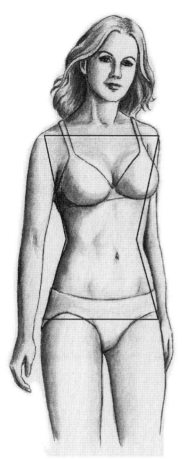

IDEAL

This is a great shape to be in (couldn't help that pun). Your shoulders and hips are balanced and you have a well defined waistline. A woman with this shape is fortunate because she can wear almost any style and weight gain or loss is generally evenly distributed, so it will often go unnoticed for long periods of time. The only hitch is whether your proportions are out of whack which can create a bit of challenge finding clothes in the right lengths for your body's proportion. A common pattern I see with women is a long rise, but short legs in relation to the body. This conundrum can make finding great fitting pants a challenge. But in terms of your figure, consider yourself blessed if you fall into the Ideal category.

Ideal Celebrities
Jessica Alba, Jessica Biel, Jennifer Aniston, Sandra Bullock, Rihanna, Demi Moore

TRANSFORMATION IN ACTION: MEET DIANE

Diane is a 35-year-old creative arts professor at a prominent university who struggled with finding clothes to flatter her toned and muscular frame. At average height, with long red-hair and a really toned physique, she had all the makings of a woman who could turn heads. But she wasn't, because she had no idea what to wear to flatter her body. Her main challenge was pants because of her full, toned thighs. To get a proper fit, she usually ended up wearing them a size larger, but then they did not sit well on her waist. She had also been shying away from skirts and dresses. So Diane presented her image as very tomboyish—wearing too big slacks, boxy shirts and jackets and saving the few dresses she owned for cocktails. The one giveaway that she had more sass in her than her clothes suggested, was her collection of sky high heels—she loved shoes and had no problem Flaunting them.

What we discovered in Diane's consult was that she had a distorted body image. She felt her body was the culprit and that's why she could not find clothes to flatter her. But when Diane understood 1) that her figure was actually ideal 2) she had to accommodate her muscular thighs, calves and arms, but it did not mean giving up her femininity and 3) in addition to her thighs being healthy, she had an unusually long rise and short legs for her height, she was suddenly liberated from years of feeling and dressing frumpy. She no longer saw her body as the enemy, but learned the techniques to highlight her amazing assets, and more importantly learned to embrace her muscular thighs. This was a huge 'aha' for her. She learned that lower rise pants with a tab waist front and stretch in the fabric most flattered her. And skirts and dresses became her new friends, as I helped her see that her lower legs were an incredible asset (so shapely!) that needed to be Flaunted.

If you catch Diane now, she is most likely in a waist cinching dress just above her knee with her fabulous heels and newfound love for bangles. She is a woman who gets noticed with her chic red blow out and signature style. She embraces her femininity and is no longer afraid to show off her amazing figure. She learned the art of figure flattering and looks simply fabulous.

Observation: *Learning the art of figure flattery is like learning anything else. It takes time, patience, and effort, but once you get it, it can totally transform the way you look and the way you view clothes. For Diane, knowing that she was not alone in her figure challenge was a huge relief, along with knowing her issue could be addressed. Often, women internalize their body issues and don't know where to go for help. They, like Diane, think their bodies are at fault somehow. I hope you learn from this chapter that your body is never wrong. You just have to be armed with the tools to dress it right.*

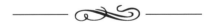

TRIANGLE

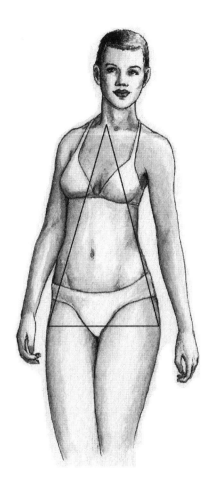

The triangle shaped woman is wider in the hips than the shoulders. The triangle is often called "pear shaped" and is the most common shape. Women who are triangular have full thighs and bottoms with narrow shoulders and smaller bust lines. Their hips are full and often tapered, which means the widest part is further down their frames toward the top of their legs.

The challenge for triangle shaped women is that when clothes fit around the hip area, they need to be taken in at the waist. Because of her comparatively narrower shoulders, her figure appears bottom heavy.

Let's have a look at the most flattering styles for a triangular shape.

Slacks

The very womanly pear shaped figure is best suited to tailored slacks that:

- Sit slightly below the natural waistline so as not to accentuate the curve between the waist and hips;

- Don't have side pockets, pleats, gathers or any detailing near the hip;

- Fall from the widest part of the hip or thigh in a straight line or with a slight flare from the knee;

- Are made from soft, draping fabrics that fall beautifully;

- Are darker in color than the top so she looks visually slimmer on her bottom half;

- Are in fabrics that accommodate the curves—usually slacks with 2% lycra or spandex will help. Also look for pants with a higher rise in the back to accommodate the tush;

- Utilize vertical seams, ribbing or stripes in the fabric; and

- Are not tapered or straight cut pants, as these will accentuate the hips and thighs and emphasize her bottom heaviness.

Dresses & Skirts

When it comes to dresses and skirts—whether casual or cocktail - let's look at the styles that best work for this shape and those that don't.

- The essential thing is to look for dresses that add volume or detail on top while draping over the hips (rather than clinging).

- A-line dresses and skirts will skim over those hips and minimize their width.

- Dresses and skirts that fall to the knee, with fullness or flounce are very flattering as they balance the hips.

- V shaped or wide scoop necklines emphasize the top part of this body type and widen the shoulders so the hips appear more balanced.

- Dresses and skirts with vertical seaming or stripes will flatter this shape.

- Avoid horizontal details near the hips, which make them look wider.

- Avoid stiff fabrics with no give, which do not accommodate fuller hips thighs and rear.

Jackets and Tops

When looking for tops and jackets, the goal is to add structure and width around your shoulder and upper torso to balance your wider hips.

- In a jacket or coat, look for shoulder pads and wider lapels.

- Have fun with color and striking necklines to employ "eyes up".

- Details like puffed sleeves, shoulder epaulets or boatnecks will make your shoulders appear wider, thereby making you look more balanced.

- Avoid dainty collars and unstructured shoulders, which make the shoulders look narrower.

- Skinny lapels, narrow V necks and crew neck styles will only further narrow your shoulder, so avoid them.

- Wear jackets and tops that either sit at the narrower part of your hips or those that end higher, just below your natural waist. This is to avoid your tops ending where you are widest, so you are not overly emphasizing your hips.

Triangle Celebrities
Beyonce, Michelle Obama, Hillary Clinton, Kate Winslet, Julianna Margulies, Kristin Davis, America Ferrera

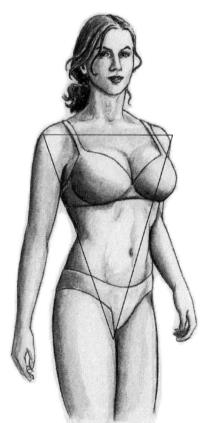

INVERTED TRIANGLE

The inverted triangle or 'strawberry' shaped woman has wide, strong shoulders and narrower hips, tush and thighs. She tends to have a full bust with a broad back and long, shapely legs. Her challenge is that when clothes fit her waist, they are often too full in the hips. Her main goal is to balance her wide shoulders with her narrow hips, otherwise she may appear top heavy.

Slacks
Inverted triangles tend to have great legs, but finding the perfect pair of tailored pants can be challenging because the hips are so narrow. Typically, I advise women with this figure type to highlight their gorgeous legs with skirts and dresses. Still, if you're willing to do the leg work, the most flattering pants for you will have these qualities:

- Be tailored so they fall in a straight line from the hip;

- Include details like side or flap pockets that add extra dimension to your hips;

- Include horizontal details or seaming around the hip area;

- Have texture or be of heavier fabric, both which add more bulk to your hips to balance your wider shoulders. Fabrics that hold their shape like linen or corduroy are good for you;

- Be mid-tone to lighter colors, so you bring more attention to your hips and thighs; and

- Fit the thighs or else you'll wind up looking bigger than you really are.

Dresses & Skirts
The goal with dresses is to emphasize your great legs with simple bodices and full skirts. Suggestions:

- A fitted bodice with a softly flared skirt gives you balance;

- Trendy one shoulder dresses or halter styles visually narrow your shoulders while also showing them off. Just be sure to wear a supportive bra;

- You can wear a shift/sheath dress as long as the fabric has "give" to accommodate your wide back, and the neckline is a deep narrow V or scoop; and

- Bias cut skirts or dresses will flatter your hips because they will hug them while flaring out at the knee. Any skirts or dresses with volume on the bottom really bring your shoulders into balance.

Avoid the following:

- Off the shoulder or boat neck necklines or any accents like puff sleeves or shoulder padded dresses that call attention to your shoulders;

- Very fitted or pencil skirts which make you look too top heavy; and

- Wearing skirts and dresses way past your knees which hides your killer legs.

Jackets & Tops

Inverted triangle shapes look good in belted jackets that create more volume below the waist without overemphasizing the shoulders. The cutest jackets and tops are:

- Styles that flare from the waist in a peplum style;

- Those with small lapels and no shoulder pads;

- Designs that accommodate and contour over your full bust-line;

- Those with asymmetrical, one shoulder, halter and other necklines that showcase your shoulders while visually making them appear narrower; and

- Single button jackets, that make you look slimmer through the torso.

Styles to avoid include:

- Double breasted styles which make you look top heavy;

- Wide lapels, shoulder pads and epaulettes;

- Over-accessorizing with scarves, brooches or necklaces, which draw too much attention to your top; and

- Cropped jackets with slim fitting bottoms.

Inverted Triangle Celebrities

Vanessa Williams, Bo Derek, Angelina Jolie, Catherine Zeta-Jones, Tina Turner, Sherri Shepherd

HOURGLASS

During the 1950s and early 1960s, every woman wanted to have an hourglass figure and attempted to do so with heavy corseting.

The hourglass woman has wide shoulders and a full bosom, with high hips that are balanced to her shoulders. She generally has curvy thighs, and her trademark is a very defined waist—usually more than 10 inches smaller than her hips.

The challenge for the hourglass woman is finding clothes that contour with her feminine curves, otherwise she can look much larger than she really is.

Slacks

The hourglass shaped woman is usually pretty well balanced top and bottom. The struggle with finding a stylish pair of tailored slacks is getting them to fit her tiny waist while still fitting her curvy hips. Some tips:

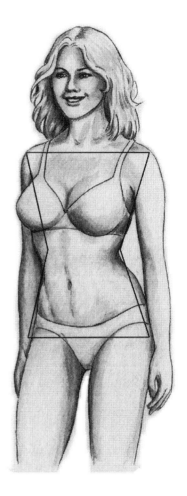

- You can't go wrong with wide legged trousers in a soft fabric;

- Mid rise pants that flare from the hip step up your style;

- Try boot cut style pants to balance you out on the bottom;

- Look for slacks in fabrics that accommodate your curves. Usually, slacks with 2% Lycra or spandex will do the trick;

- Look for pants with a higher rise in the back, but that contour lower in the front. Styles built for curvy frames are your friend;

- Avoid slouchy, baggy styles; and

- Stay away from details like side pockets that over-exaggerate your hips.

Dresses & Skirts

The heavenly hourglass shape was just made for dresses, so have some fun.

- Stick to styles that highlight your waist.

- Wrap dresses that tie at the front or back will highlight that waist.

- Scoop necks, sweetheart and V necklines all accentuate your bust while visually trimming your waist.

- Shaped strapless dresses can work as long as they are structured to add support to your bust line.

- Look for styles with side ruching that also highlight the waist and contour with your curves.

- Empire waists and sheath styles don't do your figure any favors.

Avoid:

- Frills and bows on the bodice if you have a large bust; and

- Tight skirts if you're heavy on the bottom.

Jackets & Tops

Structure will define and silhouette your shape, so aim for more tailored tops and jackets that are nipped in at the waist.

- Belted tops and jackets were made for you!

- Jackets and tops with princess seaming contour nicely over your curves. The peplum jacket with its nipped in waist will flatter you amazingly.

- Jackets that button under the bust (lower stance) look great.

- Long V necks help elongate your torso and flatter your bust line, but avoid wide lapels.

- Avoid shapeless, slouchy or boxy styles.

Hourglass Celebrities
Sophia Loren, Selma Hayek, Marilyn Monroe, Halle Berry, Kim Kardashian, Oprah, Sofia Vergara.

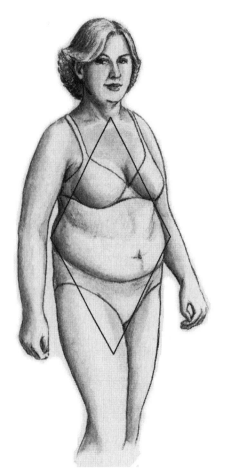

ROUND OR DIAMOND

Round shaped women tend to have the same proportions across the shoulders as they do across the hips with a prominent mid section, including the waist and tummy areas. They are usually short waisted.

The challenge for round shaped women is elongating and slimming the body and minimizing the tummy area.

Slacks
Although you may have slim legs, showing them off in figure hugging pants will only draw attention to your ample mid-section. Instead here are a few slack style solutions.

- Choose classic shapes that are flat fronted with no pleats or gathering.

- Pants should sit comfortably just below the waist. Avoid too tight waistbands.

- Slacks should drape smoothly to the ankle in soft fabrics that don't cling.

- Look for styles with classic widths or wider to help you balance out your middle. If you're tall, you can try palazzo styles in fabrics with substantial drape.

- Boot cut style pants with higher rises will flatter you the best. Avoid low rise styles which will essentially give you two tummy bulges.

54

- You will definitely need to look for the curvy fit styles for the most comfortable fit.

- Look for very plain pants with minimal details. But do look for pockets in the back as they can detract from a large tush.

- Accentuate your black slacks (dark slacks are your new friends) with black pointy heels. This lengthens the leg line and makes you look taller and slimmer.

- Stay away from slouchy, baggy pants as these styles do nothing for you.

Dresses & Skirts

To capture the glow of rosy round shapes, accentuate the neckline or hem with some razzle-dazzle to draw attention away from the middle section.

- Empire waist dresses with ¾ length sleeves are figure flattering.

- Flared maxi dresses that fall from under the bust look good and help you look taller and slimmer. Just avoid overly busy or large prints.

- A low-cut V neckline visually slims and elongates you.

- Choose substantial fabrics that drape your body, but don't cling.

- Look for wide, sweetheart or boat neck necklines to widen the shoulder line so your tummy looks smaller by comparison.

- Asymmetrical patterns/diagonal lines are wonderful to detract and keep the focus where you want it.

- Draping or ruching can be wonderfully slimming if they're in the right spots and in good quality fabrics.

- Always do "eyes up"—wear substantial accessories that match your frame and capture attention at your neck and above.

- Steer clear of any detailing or belts around the waist area.

- Stay away from shapeless shift dresses.

Jackets and Tops

Streamline your shape with tops that camouflage your middle. Here are a few suggestions:

- A structured hip length jacket elongates your line, especially if you wear it open;

- A boxy tweed jacket will be very forgiving in the cooler months and is a classic staple;

- A loosely fitted wrap shirt is very figure flattering and can camouflage a tummy effectively;

- Layering will serve you well. Use a thinner dark layer under a jacket for a slimming look;

- Long V necks and nipped in waists add definition;

- Try a classic trench or topper jacket with a defined shoulder line and wear it open for pizzazz with slacks; and

- Stay away from boxy, shapeless jackets that end at the waist and leave the tummy exposed.

Round Celebrities
Rosie O'Donnell, Aretha Franklin, Roseanne Barr, Gabourney Sidibe

RECTANGLE

The rectangular woman has a balanced shoulder and hip line with no defined waist. She tends to be small breasted with few curves, an angular body and usually she has long legs.

The challenge for rectangles is finding ways to add curves to the silhouette. They usually have to let out the waistbands on their off-the-rack clothing.

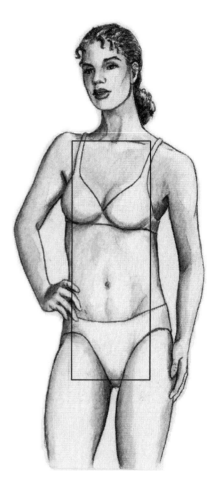

Slacks

Rectangular or boyish silhouettes were made to wear classic slacks in a wide variety of styles. Try the following:

- High waisted wide leg pants with a stylish belt to create a waistline;

- Slim fitting straight legged pants with a tuxedo stripe to add texture;

- Boot cut style pants to add curves;

- Pants with side seam pockets or hip pockets to create the illusion of curves;

- Pants with a gentle flare from the knee to add dimension; and

- Skinny jeans if you are slender.

Dresses & Skirts

Most dresses will look fine on a rectangle shaped woman, but for more of a wow factor, you need to add some womanly curves. Here are some style tips for you.

- Bias cut dresses/skirts give you real "ooh la la".

- Bows or sashes at the waist or hip add contours.

- Look for contouring details in the design or pattern. Princess seams are your really good friends because they do just that.

- A-line skirts and dresses add needed curves.

- Ruffles, tiers and flounces add softness to your angles.

- Dresses and skirts should end at the knee with lots of volume.

- Fitted tops with a flared skirt, create the illusion of a waist and are very flattering.

- Halter necks with flare (and flair) look great on you.

- Avoid vertical patterns or lines which just make you look straighter.

- Straight sheath dresses won't do you any favors so avoid as well.

Jackets & Tops
Structured coats and jackets look great, but your boyish shape needs extra accents to add more figure flattery. Suggestions:

- A shawl collar wrap style jacket or blouse;

- Defined waist accents, such as the corseted blazer or peplum style which gives you maximum curve appeal;

- Tops with princess seaming to visually add curves;

- An empire waist style with a very wide or sweetheart neckline to bypass the waist altogether; and

- Sharp, structured jackets that add curves.

Avoid:
- Slouchy or boyfriend jackets; and

- Boxy or tubular jackets without belts.

Rectangle Celebrities
Cameron Diaz, Heidi Klum, Kate Hudson, Naomi Campbell, Gwyneth Paltrow

BLENDED SHAPE

While a majority of women fall pretty much into one of the 6 main shape categories, there is certainly a cross section that does not. Some women have a blended shape, which usually means they will have one or two distinctive features that make them "non-standard".

As an example, a woman may be a rectangle shape, but she has a larger than standard bust. Or a woman who is a classic inverted triangle may have a large tummy that makes the width of her hips appear wider.

The trick is to work with the predominant shape category that mirrors your body's shape and then make adjustments for your unique features by following the above guidelines. Enhance the features that are your best and camouflage the features you want to disguise.

ARE YOU LONG LEGGED OR SHORT WAISTED?

Proportion is another element in determining how great you look in your clothing. It relates to the verticality in your body and how different aspects including your torso, rise, upper and lower legs relate to each other and whether they are in proportion relative to your height. This is an important point. Your figure and proportions are distinct and unique to you. When you understand how to dress your figure coupled with your body's proportions, it is the *"je ne sais quoi"* that separates the women who look fabulous from the one just looking okay.

Have you ever gone on a shopping spree only to find that the pair of tailored black slacks which looked stunning on the rack, make your crotch area look like a sack of potatoes; or that the gorgeous chartreuse cocktail dress "sort-of" fits, except the waistband sits too high or low on your body? Those are proportion (not figure) issues.

Herein lies the real challenge. Most designers work from a standard template (a fit model); so it doesn't take much logic to realize that the pattern created from the designers' fit model may not work for your figure type. THEN, add the fact that the same fit model may have proportions that are way different from yours. She may have a shorter torso or longer legs. Suppose you have a long torso or short legs? Do you see the fit conundrum? That designer's garments are not going to fit your body well. And, you have no way of knowing this until you try the garment on.

Quite frankly, designers often design for their ideal client (who is typically a size 2 fashionista who may have little in common with you); so if you find off-the-rack garments that work their magic on you, it is a godsend. (Which is why we talk later on about the importance of making friends with a tailor or seamstress.)

But don't get discouraged. Stay with me here.

While you can't do anything to alter the body proportions you were born with, you can absolutely use tactics to visually elongate or shorten areas of your body so it appears more proportioned. And therein lies one of the little known *secrets* to appearing taller, more proportioned and absolutely fabulous!

Often when I share these tricks with women they are amazed at 1) how easy and simple they are, and 2) how great the impact is. All it takes is a little education and that is what I am going to share with you.

To balance your figure and proportions, there are two rules you need to commit to memory. **RULE #1:** Where you are short, you want to visually lengthen and where you are long you want to visually shorten.

RULE #2: Horizontal lines, patterns or details shorten and widen. Vertical lines, patterns or details lengthen and slim.

If you *just* remember these two rules, you are well on your way to dressing in ways that make you look balanced and proportioned.

Without getting into too much detail here, you can quickly determine whether your legs are long or short for your body, so you'll know where you need to visually lengthen or shorten.

Do this simple exercise: Measure the area from your crotch to the floor with a measuring tape. This is actually your inseam measurement. You'll want to note this number for future reference when ordering pants online. Then take your height in inches and subtract the inseam measurement from it. This second measurement is essentially

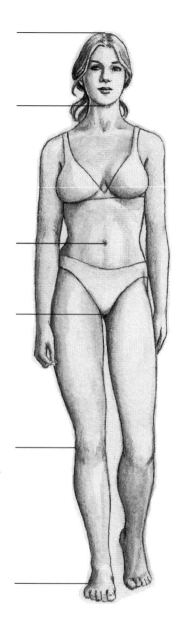

the length of your upper body, as the body is technically cut in half at the crotch area. Which number is larger? If your inseam measurement is larger it means your legs are long for your body. If the upper body measurement is larger, it could indicate a long torso or a long rise (the area from your waist to your crotch).

Let's use an example. Mary's inseam is 32". She is 5' 6" which equates to 66". 66-32=34". In Mary's case, her legs are 2 inches short for her height. If she were proportioned top to bottom, her measurements would be even; 33"/33". Because the top half of her body is 2 inches longer, the extra inches could be because her torso/rise is long. In Mary's case, she would be trying to put her body in proportion by using tactics to visually lengthen her legs by at least 2 inches. An easy fix is for her to wear 2 inch heels. With that she gets the extra 2 inches in her legs to make it proportioned to her body.

See how straightforward this all turns out to be once you understand the mystery behind your body particulars? I trust this is all coming together for you and making a whole lot of sense. Perhaps you've even had an "aha" or two by now about why certain pieces fit you amazingly and why others look just awful. It's not just the luck of the draw. There are reasons for your slam dunks and your kaputs, and now you should be crystal clear about how to create more slam dunks with your clothing. You just have to understand your body and learn how to dress to enhance it. Now isn't that liberating!

10 Tips TO LOOK TALLER, SLIMMER AND MORE POISED IN 10 MINUTES

Let's face it. Most women want to look taller and slimmer. So to make this REALLY effortless for you, I've compiled a list of tactics (some we may have already discussed), that all help you appear taller and slimmer overall. With your understanding of your own figure and a sense of your legs in relation to your torso, you can use these tips to create the illusion of a slimmer, taller you. I hope you're already starting to feel really excited to learn these tips and tricks and put them to work in your wardrobe. Without further ado, I present: 10 Tips to Look Taller, Slimmer and More Poised in 10 minutes.

1. **Show off your upper chest**. Banish those dowdy baggy turtlenecks from your closet and add tops with V necks, or wide scoop necklines. When you show off your upper chest (and even a little cleavage if you're comfortable doing that), it creates a focal point away from any figure flaws below and creates the illusion of a longer slimmer you. The deeper the plunge of the top or shirt, the more the narrowest part of it hones in on the waist, making it look smaller as well. A great way to execute this look is to wear a jacket with a low stance below the bust (very deep plunge) and wear a cami in a lively color under it. Your waist will look smaller and your overall look will appear slimmer and taller.

2. **Go for monochromatic dressing**. Wearing the same or varying shades of the same color from top to bottom is extremely elongating. If the colors happen to be dark, they will be slimming as well. Be clear: monochromatic does not mean only dressing in all black! It simply means wearing one primary hue, or tonal variations of the same hue, from top to bottom so you have one long uninterrupted line of color, which creates verticality in your body. Picture a pastel pink blouse, with ivory slacks, and light beige shoes and see how this can be somewhat monochromatic because the contrasts in the colors are very slight? Or imagine an olive skirt suit paired with an emerald green cami and dark grey shoes. Still monochromatic. Or you can wear a chocolate brown dress with tall chocolate brown boots paired with brown tights and be absolutely monochromatic, tall and slim. Get the picture? Or go monochromatic on your bottom half only, to elongate your legs. Wear stockings/tights that blend with the color

of your shoes and/or hemline where possible. In the summer, wear nude shoes to match your skin tone for the same elongating effect.

3. If you want to look tall and slim, **look for vertical lines in print, pattern or construction** in your ensembles. Vertical lines can be created with princess seams, zippers, scarves, open jackets or cardigans—truly anything that encourages the eye to move up and down. This visually creates a slimmer silhouette. A navy pinstriped pants suit is a great example of this tactic. A V neck knee length dress with vertical seaming details from top to bottom will have a similar effect.

4. **Use the principle of "eyes up"** by using your accessories strategically. For example, a long, oblong scarf in one of your "wow" colors worn over a jacket can have a slimming, elongating effect. Long necklaces can act like a plunging neckline in that they create a deep 'V' in the front of the body, taking attention away from your hips and drawing it to your front and waistline. The deep V tactic also elongates the neck, an instant height enhancer. Big dangly earrings draw the eyes of the onlooker to your face and not your middle where you may be carrying extra pounds.

5. **Wear your hair up and away from your face**. This is a simple trick that easily adds height if you create volume in the crown and wear your hair in a high pony tail or chic chignon. Wearing your hair pulled back also helps highlight your cheekbones and forehead, all which can make your face look thinner.

6. **Wear the highest heel that is comfortable for you** and get it in a pointy toe version. Legs look slim and toned in heels with a tapered front and heels of course add height. Avoid ankle strap shoes that can actually interrupt the long line of the leg and ankle.

7. **Get rid of capri pants** that end at the calf, especially those that flare out. They are instant leg shorteners and make women look frumpy. Pants with cuffed bottoms also chop off the leg line. A cuffed capri pant is not your friend if you want to look tall and svelte.

8. **Wear ¾ length sleeves**. This is one of those optical illusions that just works. Try it in the mirror—scrunch up or (as I like to say to clients) "juuge" your sleeves up and see what happens to your legs (hint: it makes them look longer). When I show clients this trick in the mirror they are always amazed.

9. **Don a topper jacket that hits you below your hips worn open.** This is a great figure camouflaging tactic if you have wide hips, a big tush or full thighs. The straight lines of the jacket worn open over a blouse, Tee or cami, work to counteract and hide excess curves, making you look slimmer and taller.

10. **Invest in the best bra you can afford.** The right fitting bra can shave off 10 pounds and give you better posture, as your breasts are supported and lifted and your torso is elongated by the extra space this creates. Shapewear, as in panty shapers and the likes, smoothes out bulges and creates a sleeker profile in your clothes so you look more streamlined, slimmer and taller. Shapewear is your friend, ladies. Spanx anyone?

BECOMING FABULOUS

1. Take a good hard look at yourself in the mirror and choose *at least 10 things* about your body you LOVE. Make a note of them if you have to so you don't forget!

2. Determine which of the 6 body shapes you fit and choose a celebrity or someone you admire with a similar body shape whose style of dressing you can emulate.

3. Just for fun, put together a scrapbook with your favorite looks that suit your body shape so you can use them as inspiration when you're shopping for new clothes.

Chapter Four

Factoring for Fit

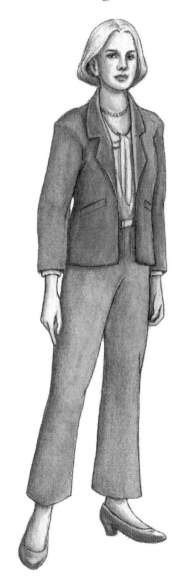

Steps to Flaunting it

✔ Don't think you're all on your own when you can't find off the rack clothes that fit. It's a very common problem. Once you understand and make friends with your unique body shape, you can train your eye to instantly recognize which styles are going to be most flattering.

✔ Find a quality tailor or seamstress who will help alter your clothes to get the right fit. Once you accept that finding the perfect fit in ready to wear clothing is more the exception than the rule, you will feel so much happier about going shopping.

✔ If you are a petite, tall or plus-sized, carefully study the stylist secrets included in this chapter so you can dress to flatter your figure.

In the last chapter, we discussed the 6 basic figure types, so now you know which body shape mirrors your own and you can highlight your assets and look fabulous!

We are now going to address tailoring and fit so that everything you own and wear fits you to a "T". No more standing at the closet door frustrated because nothing in your wardrobe fits well. In this chapter, we will also discuss the harder to fit statures—petites, talls and plus, and how to pull your look effortlessly together—regardless of your challenges—so you always look smashing.

By the end of this chapter, you'll want to race to your closet every morning with a huge smile on your face because you *know* that the clothes in your closet fit you as though they were personally tailored just for your body. And that is just how it should be.

FIT FIXES

Working to get the right fit comes with the territory if you want your clothes to flatter you. It's time to stop kvetching when you find a gorgeous pair of black evening slacks that are perhaps too long in the crotch or too long, period.

If the waist band fits snugly and is where the waist band should be, if the slacks hug you just right around your tush and fall beautifully, and if the vertical seaming elongates your legs and hides your tummy bulge, then you have found the ideal pair of pants. A clever tailor (which we'll be chatting about real soon) can quickly make the necessary length adjustments to customize to your leg length.

As you make friends with your body shape and understand the styles that best suit it, you'll learn to train your eyes to instantly recognize the cuts and styles that flatter your figure.

Although it's generally assumed that quality labels and designers are automatically going to provide you with the perfect fit, that's not always the case. Sure, quality garments are more likely to result in a better all-around fit, but high-end designers use a variety of templates to cut their patterns, and those templates may not bear any resemblance to your particular body.

It pays to find which designer brands and styles work for your body shape and then stick with them. If you do strike it lucky and find a perfect pair of slacks, buy three of them. Seriously! If it comes in different colors, even better. Pants are one of the hardest clothing items to find a perfect fit, so indulge yourself when you find a pair that flatters you. Plus, no one's going to notice you're wearing the same slacks, especially if you mix and match with varying tops and accessories. It will be your little secret.

Let's have a look at some of the key elements for a perfect fit.

- **Jackets:** The shoulders should line up with your hips. Unless you are looking for an elongated jacket (which goes in and out of fashion), the hem should generally extend no further than the tips of your fingers.

  The armholes should be wide enough to fit the top of your arms comfortably without pulling or puckering. The sleeves should hit at wrist bone level or slightly above if you want to show off bracelets and jewelry.

  Jackets with ¾ length sleeves are very on-trend too. If the jacket fits well else-where but is short in the sleeves, simply have the sleeve adjusted (or roll them up) so it falls midway between your wrist and elbow.

  Jacket Test: Fold your arms across your chest. Is the jacket comfortable across your back? Does it strain or sag at the shoulders? Button all the buttons on the jacket to make sure they are secure, and don't pull. Buttonholes should be neatly stitched so they don't fray. Most quality designers include at least one extra button. Make sure the jacket fits you well buttoned up and there is no gaping or pulling.

- **Pants**: Pants should fit on your high hip depending on how long the rise is. Nowadays, most slacks fit at or just below your belly button, unless you're trying on low rise pants. If you have a good fit at the waistband, you will not need to keep pulling your pants up. If your pants ride down on you constantly, it is a sign that it's a poor fit—either a waistband that is too loose, a rise too long or a pant that is too big on you overall.

  When trying on pants, make sure you wear the shoes you intend to be wearing with them. Bend your knees and squat to make sure the crotch isn't too tight or short. You really want to get a perfect fit in the crotch area. The crotch (or rise) of a pant is too short for you if it pulls and wrinkles at the side of the crotch, especially when you walk. The crotch is too long for you when it sags and leaves a pool of fabric settled unattractively at the crotch when you're seated. Both of these are deal breakers.

If the pants have side pockets, they should lie against your hipline without gaping or pulling. If the pockets gape open, the pants are too tight or the pockets are too low. If they only gape at the pockets and otherwise fit fine, you can have your new best friend, your tailor, stitch the pockets shut.

The correct length should clear the heel of your shoes and rest on the front part of your foot with a small break between the hem and the shoe.

- **Skirts**: The hemline of a skirt should finish at the most flattering part of your leg, which for many women is at or slightly above the knee. It's important to examine your leg's length and shape to determine the most flattering length.

Unless the skirt has an asymmetrical hemline, the hem should fall evenly all the way around. If the skirt hikes up in the back, it's because you likely have a generous tush. This is a fit issue.

A slim-line pencil skirt can be tapered to follow the natural line of the leg. With a pencil skirt, be sure you can sit in it without it riding up or pulling at the sides. Also make sure when you walk, the skirt does not start to bunch up on the sides—a sign that your hips are too wide or your rear too pronounced to accommodate the straightness in this skirt style.

A-line skirts gently flare out from the hip. Just ensure that the skirt isn't too wide or bulky on your frame. The fabric should fall gracefully over your legs.

TAILOR MADE

As the proud owner of a slender, 6' 1" frame, and a lover of clothes that make me look and feel fabulous, I've grown quite accustomed to becoming acquainted with a number of professional tailors. I've learned to accept that when I buy clothes off the rack, 7 times out of 10 they have to be altered, so having a professional tailor or seamstress as part of my team of service providers is a must.

One of the most common stories I hear from my clients is, "I can never find anything that fits," so don't think you're all on your own if that's part of your story too. Most women believe they should be able to buy all their clothing off the rack and have it fit perfectly, but sadly that's not the case. Whether you are petite, tall, boyish, full figured or plus sized, the reality is that you are lucky if you find something that fits perfectly right out of the gate.

Let's face facts: the first is learning to embrace your stature and the figure and size you are now. The second is understanding that in all likelihood you will need to alter ready to wear clothes. Once you accept these two facts, then you will take your clothes to get altered as a matter of course and not think twice about it. Shopping becomes a pleasure because you are armed with the tools that help you understand how you can achieve a fabulous look with just minor sewing fixes.

It's important to find a tailor or seamstress that understands almost as well as you do your unique body shape and knows how to make the correct alterations to get the fit just right. As you would when seeking any professional, shop around.

SIZING UP YOUR STATURE: PETITES, TALLS, PLUS-SIZED

Now that you have a better sense of how to dress to flatter your figure, what's next? We are going to take a look at making the most of your stature so you sizzle. Whether you're petite, tall or plus size, finding clothes that fit impeccably can be challenging, but if you pay attention to the style secrets I'm about to uncover, you can rock your look, no matter what your frame. And who better can relate to you than a 6 feet tall woman?

Polished Petites
Petite women are generally recognized as being 5'2" or shorter and smaller in overall

proportions. They tend to have narrower shoulders, shorter arms and legs and less distance from their necks to their waists than their taller counterparts.

The secret to presenting a polished petite image, is using line and proportion to visually elongate the body. This can be achieved by creating a vertical, unbroken line in your silhouette that moves upward. Clearly the most important goal for the petite woman is appearing taller. If you are petite, here are a few great strategies you can use:

- ❖ The most obvious tactic is to wear the highest heel you can while still feeling comfortable. The operative word here is "comfortable", so if 2 inches is your limit, so be it.

- ❖ Choose monochromatic ensembles with no obvious breaks, such as a wide belt or waist panel in a different color. Every time you create a "break" in color, the eye will stop at the color change which in effect creates a horizontal line. If you are paying attention and remembering our rules, this will make you appear even shorter. As we mentioned in the last chapter, monochromatic doesn't necessarily mean the exact same color; it can mean a soft pink blouse with cream slacks or a heather gray sweater and black skirt, or it can mean a teal suit. Slight color variations are fine. However, the more contrast in your outfit, the less monochromatic it will be, and the more the horizontal lines created by the contrasting colors will "break" your length, making you look shorter (and wider).

- ❖ Look for higher waistbands in skirts and pants and then tuck your top in (if your figure allows it). This makes your legs look longer which makes you look taller.

- ❖ Choose clothing with a focus on vertical lines and details. Accents like pin-stripes, princess seams, vertical seams, ribbed knits or corduroy that runs vertically all add length.

- ❖ A petite woman can really benefit by focusing on higher necklines or turtle neck styles because this adds height to your frame (again if these are figure flattering silhouettes for you).

- ❖ Zoom in on details like a long row of buttons on a sweater or vertical piping on a jacket, all which elongate your torso.

- ❖ Look for ¾ length sleeves which optically make legs look longer.

❖ Avoid clothing that is too busy, voluminous, fussy or with a strong pattern. These design elements overwhelm your small frame.

❖ Stay away from cropped pants—they are the ultimate leg shortener.

❖ If you want to wear cuffed pants, ensure your stockings and shoes match the color of the pants to continue the uninterrupted vertical line.

❖ You can get away with large prints as long as they are in muted or low contrast colors.

❖ Skirts that fall just above the knee give you the longest length, but if you choose to wear a longer skirt, keep the fabric light and look for skirts that are tapered to follow the natural curves of your body. To disguise large calves, make sure the skirt falls below the heaviest part of your lower leg.

❖ Create interest around your face by employing "eyes up" (Yes, I know we've mentioned this repeatedly in this book—it's because it really works!). Accessories are a terrific way to emphasize your face and they can also help create a long line. Wear long necklaces or an oblong scarf draped loosely over an outfit. To keep the focus on your face, choose small earrings that pick up a color from the scarf or match the colors in the necklace.

TRANSFORMATION IN ACTION:
MEET DEBBY

Debby is a busy professional in her mid 40's. She is 5'1"—a classic petite and a size 6. She has a triangular build. Debby holds a senior VP position with many people reporting to her and she needs to project command, confidence and authority. Moreover, she needs to be a positive role model for her junior reports. Debby however, is stuck in an image rut. She has been wearing the same "uniform" for decades—clothing that is no longer stylish, does not fit or flatter her petite frame, and that makes her look dowdy and older than she needs to. Her closet is filled with pants suits with very long jackets. Since she does not like wearing heels, she looks shorter than her height warrants. Debby needed to work with her proportions (her legs were short for her body) and her triangular figure to create looks that made her look taller and more authoritative.

We added skirt suits in her "wow" colors to her wardrobe, paired with very structured jackets to give her the physical presence she needed. The skirts were hemmed, so they fit right at her knee to show off her shapely long lower legs; and the jackets were no longer than just below her hips. We made sure the jacket sleeves were altered so that her wrists no longer were smothered in too much fabric. Even though we tried to find most of her clothes in petites, when we couldn't, we adjusted them accordingly. The extra money spent getting clothes altered paid off in untold dividends. Debby looked better than ever after her closet overhaul and gained much needed confidence about her look. She transformed to a petite with panache and took 10 years off her look.

Observation: *When clothes fit us poorly, we feel poorly too. We may not know what is off but we know we are barely hitting the ball, far less knocking it out of the park. When we wear clothes that flatter and fit, our confidence soars and those around us can see the difference. We are validated by our new look because of the compliments we get. We walk differently and may behave differently. The transformation trickles over into other areas of our life. It is life changing.*

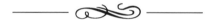

Talls that Turn Heads

From my experiences working with a variety of women, most of them envy tall women and think we have an easy time finding clothes to fit and flatter our long frames. However, I assure you, it's not so! Tall women have to get really resourceful to make our ensembles work. The greatest challenge for talls is finding clothes that are cut long enough because pants, skirts, jacket sleeves and waistbands in dresses are invariably too short for our frames.

Let's look at some style secrets for tall women:

❖ I love my svelte, statuesque frame but I don't want to be mistaken for a bean pole. One of the strategies I use is what I call, 'breaking up my height'. What this means is that I literally truncate my body via layers and accessories, so instead of one long, uninterrupted line, you see several (the exact opposite of what a petite woman wants to do). As an example, I'll wear a hip length jacket with a contrasting colored longer layer underneath, slim jeans and brown knee high boots. With this ensemble, I have created 4 horizontal lines across my body which makes me appear less linear.

Or, I may pair a fitted shirt with a wide cinching belt in a bold color and a knee length skirt. I often work with mid- high contrast colors in my outfits to further "break" the linear look (a petite woman's fashion no-no) and rarely do monochromatic looks, unless I add a belt or accessory to break up the color.

As a fellow tall woman, you'll want to replicate this technique of breaking up your height.

❖ Look for pants with a generous seam allowance that allows them to be let out and lengthened. Also, look for pants with longer inseams. (This is when you'll find your tailor a valuable resource.)

❖ If you find jeans that you love, but they don't have enough allowance to lengthen, try tucking them into a pair of boots. Voila! Problem solved. Make sure the jeans don't buckle or you'll look like you're wearing jodhpurs. This means they must fit snugly through the hips, knees and lower leg. Using this trick, no one has to know your pants are 2" short on you (assuming you keep your boots on of course).

❖ Skirt lengths are more forgiving. A skirt that hits an average height woman just below her knee will generally hit a tall woman above her knee, so the answer is, rock *that* look! Calf length skirts may hit a tall woman just at the knee, so use your long legs to your advantage. My point is, don't fuss over skirt lengths; allow yourself to be resourceful because you can generally carry any length with style.

❖ You will often need to get *very creative* with jackets because the sleeves are never long enough. I scour the stores for jackets that are designed with ¾ length sleeves and don't worry about where the sleeves end. Cap sleeved jackets or short sleeved jackets, are of course, excellent choices.

❖ With long sleeved jackets, which will generally be short on you, you have 3 choices:

    o   Try to get the sleeve lengthened if there is enough fabric;

    o   Wear a long sleeved Tee or blouse underneath to fill the gap and to trick the eye;

○ Push or roll the sleeves up so they sit higher up your arm. This looks really cool with the right jacket, such as the casual boyfriend styles.

❖ A word on belted garments or dresses with waistbands. These are tricky because as a tall woman you will often find the waist band hits you too high. But there are ways around this. Here's an insider secret: trick the eye! Today I'm wearing a jacket that came with its own belt that hits me under the bust—not quite the right spot. So I removed the belt, cut those silly string belt loops from the sides of the jacket, and added instead one of my favorite 3-inch waist belts at my natural waist, giving me a look that totally works.

You can do the same with a jacket or a dress. Dresses with long, wrap around sashes are great because you can wrap the sash around your natural waist and tie in the front. Even where there's a visible waist seam, you can adjust the wrap to mask the seam and still have most of the sash sitting at your natural waist. No one but you will know, my tall sisters.

❖ Empire waists look great in tops; but be careful with a long empire waisted maxi dress as it will make you look even taller.

❖ Avoid overly short dresses even if you have the legs for it. On most tall women, a really short dress makes you look like you've forgotten to put your pants on. Really. Don't go more than 3 inches above the knee, particularly if you are wearing heels, because you'll start to get out of proportion very quickly.

❖ One of the dead giveaways that a tall woman is not dressing to flatter and enhance her figure is when she looks like she's wearing her little sister's clothes or she looks like she has outgrown her own clothes. This means you are wearing clothing that is visibly too short on your frame. Ladies, just don't do it—NOT a good look.

❖ Accessories can be your new best friends. Use your creative flair to create looks that enhance and add pizzazz. Layers of short and long necklaces—very fashion forward - belts of all descriptions, scarves tied in unusual and exciting ways and large totes are excellent ways to break up your height and express your personal élan. Unlike petites, you can go all out with detail on detail to break the line of your silhouette.

Plus-Sized With Panache

One of the biggest frustrations I hear from plus-sized women is the lack of variety and fashion forward clothing in their size. For years, designers have been giving this strong market segment short shrift, especially when you consider that a size 14 is the average size for US women. You would think catering to the plus-sized market would be a no-brainer, but not so. Thankfully, a few smart designers have been paying attention so you just have to do your homework.

In the meantime, these style secrets should help ease your frustration and help you find clothing that slims, contours and flatters.

- ❖ Often plus-sized women also have large busts. The most figure enhancing silhouette for a large bust is a V or scooped neckline. Open necklines are much more forgiving for you than closed ones like turtlenecks.

- ❖ Look for tops without too much detail and steer clear of voluminous looks. Instead, try tops that highlight the narrower part of your torso. Empire styles can be very flattering if they are cut just right and designed in the right fabric — not too clingy but not too heavy.

- ❖ Avoid bulky fabrics, big flap pockets, very full skirts or anything that adds unnecessary bulk. This also applies to double-breasted jackets. Layering can look great, but choose light fabrics that drape across your body.

- ❖ Look for styles that contour over your frame in fabrics with a little stretch so they give a little — "give" is really important to accommodate and move with your curves.

- ❖ If you have a tummy, try slightly longer tops with some contouring or cinching near the waist. This is critically important so you avoid a square silhouette. A peplum style jacket in a soft fabric is your best friend; it can camouflage your tummy and is very figure flattering.

- ❖ Steer clear of elastic waist bands or front pleats which only make your tummy look bigger. Flat front pants are wonderful and have the added benefit of flattening out your tummy.

- ❖ Pants should be straight or trouser width. Avoid tapered pants, capris or cropped pants as they can make you look squatter. Also, avoid skirt hemlines that hit at the widest part of your calf for the same reason.

❖ The most figure flattering look for skirts is just below the knee, especially if you have an attractive curvy lower leg.

❖ Many plus-sized women don't like showing their arms, so try a thin, stretchy knit cardigan with sleeves you can layer over sleeveless tops or dresses. Look for dresses and tops with short, ¾ length or long sleeves. The ideal length is ¾ sleeves, as they visually lengthen your legs.

❖ Avoid large, bold patterns that can make you look matronly and call attention to your size. At the same time, avoid tiny prints which look insipid on your frame.

❖ A lot of full-figured women feel they must wear black because it's a slimming color, but don't restrict yourself to an all-black wardrobe. Any dark color is flattering, so consider red, cranberry, grape, forest green, magenta, navy, brown or plum, which all look fantastic if you choose the shade that best suits your skin tone. Color adds spice and sass and much needed variety to your wardrobe.

❖ Avoid horizontal design elements like stripes, patterns, prints or seams. They will all just make you look wider.

❖ Diagonal lines are very flattering, whether they are in the construction, print, design or accents of your clothing. They also offer the gift of distraction, as the eye keeps moving to keep up with them. Imagine a long gown with diagonal tiers—very flattering.

❖ Use bold accessories for panache. Long necklaces and scarves visually lengthen your body. Brooches, earrings and bangles are fabulous and can be used strategically to draw attention away from the parts you want to disguise.

BECOMING FABULOUS

If you don't already have a professional tailor, try to find one in your area who will work with you to perfect your fit. Get recommendations from friends, colleagues or associates whose style you admire. You can bet they'll have a tailor they can suggest. If you buy clothing from higher end department stores or boutiques, they will have tailors on hand to fit you on the spot so you won't have to make an extra trip.

Chapter Five

From Plain to Polished: Developing Style

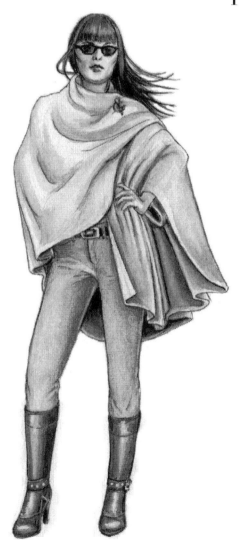

Steps to Flaunting it

🥿 Pay attention to the image you project, and the messages it conveys about you. Modify accordingly.

🥿 Using the 7 Styles as a foundation (as found in this chapter), define which of those styles most closely fits you, and then add in any additional elements that also define who you are to create a style that's yours.

🥿 Look to your fashion icons and women whose style you most admire to help you create a signature style that is uniquely yours. Use those women as inspiration to create a style that reflects the fabulous woman you are!

🥿 Be willing to allow your signature style to develop and evolve over time, as you evolve, so that it radiates the presence that is YOU.

THE STYLISH WOMAN

I'd like to revisit my business tagline: Presence With A Purpose™.

"Presence". Isn't that an interesting word? Among other things, presence is defined as *"the ability to project a sense of ease, poise, or self-assurance"*. Does that describe you? If it does, all I can say is, "You go, girl!" If not, we've got some work to do, because you won't master true presence until you have your signature style down pat.

Let's get started with a little exercise in imaginative thinking. I'd like you to imagine the following scenario, because it's likely you've experienced it at least once in your lifetime.

You catch sight of a woman in the street who immediately grabs your attention. Her hair is perfectly styled and suits the shape of her face. Her makeup is not obvious or overdone. She's outfitted with clothing that fits and flatters her silhouette, and her accessories pull together the entire ensemble for that final touch of élan.

Your 30-second 'first impression' says she is intelligent, confident, self-assured, powerful, stylish, polished and financially independent (or words to that effect), right?

On closer inspection, you may notice she is wearing a simple blouse with a black pencil skirt. But what differentiates her from the masses, is how she works that simple outfit. It's not just any blouse, but a blouse in what must be one of her power colors, because she looks radiant and vibrant, and her eyes sparkle. The blouse is simple but not boring. It has flair in the details on the sleeve, waist or collar so it looks pretty and flatters her. The skirt fits to perfection—not too snug to be seen as overtly sexy but hugging her curves artfully, so you have no doubt it's a woman's body.

Then there's the overall silhouette. Her waist may be cinched with a belt to further enhance her figure. Shoes are a knockout red, high heels of course, and high quality. But she doesn't stop there. She brings our attention back from her spectacular shoes to her face because her lips are a matching shade of red, and she may be wearing a play of red in her silk scarf.

Can you picture this woman or one like her in your mind's eye?

Note: this imaginative scenario isn't all about what she is wearing. What is equally important is her manner, poise, grace, *savoir faire* and sense of command. When she walks, she struts. This woman doesn't have to be traditionally beautiful to pull all this off. What she has instead is a keen sense of her personal style. She knows how to flatter her figure, and this gives her the confidence to Flaunt It. And all of this gives her presence.

Why is presence important? Because it conveys confidence, independence and self possession. You look like you. You're more authentic, and you're optimizing your assets to create a unique look.

All those benefits give you power—the power to use your image to your advantage.

One of the keys to having the kind of presence I just described is in knowing, understanding, defining and nailing your signature style. Tough?

It is easier than you think once you are comfortable and confident with the personal style that works for you. Sure, the imaginary woman I just described is what many of us may aspire to be; but the look that appears to have been so effortlessly pulled together has, in all probability, taken her lots of time, thought and strategy. You want to know the hard truth? Effortless style takes some effort!

IDENTIFYING YOUR PERSONAL STYLE

We've just imagined what a woman with a signature style may look like. But you might still be wondering what having style really means. In a nutshell, style is knowing who you are, embracing your unique body, and dressing in ways that look and feel best on you. Your clothing becomes just another way you express yourself and your individuality to the world. Style is about making your ensembles ring true, by mixing them with your attitude, personality and your creative use of accessories. Style is not about following fashion trends or even fashion. True style is ageless and timeless and absolutely authentic. It's about being comfortable in your skin and it's about Flaunting It.

It's all coming together now, isn't it?

One of the most important elements in my work with women is helping them discover their unique personal styles by using the seven core styles as the foundation.

The exciting part about understanding these personal styles is that with fine tuning, you begin to suss out your very own signature style. So before we go any further, let's look at highlights of each of the 7 core styles, so you can identify whether any of them says, "Hey, that sounds just like me!"

The Traditionalist

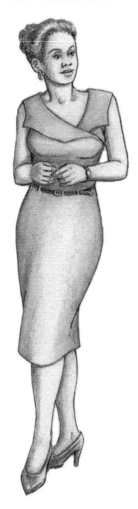

A woman who favors Traditionalist style projects a very classic, conservative and business like image that is characterized by its timelessness, durability and value. Her appearance is tasteful, well-groomed and neat.

The limiting aspects of this style are that it may appear too formal and stiff for casual occasions and too uptight for formal events. The Traditionalist woman values clothing as a personal investment in herself.

The Traditionalist's sense of style can be perceived as boring because she doesn't follow trends and is not prone to taking fashion risks. Additionally, she does not come across as soft or feminine with her choice of silhouettes and designs which veer on the practical, no-nonsense side.

Her fashion style:

- Timeless, classic, tailored and functional designs;

- Structured fit and straight hems at or below knee;

- Clean, simple lines and silhouettes are attractive to her;

- Well constructed jackets are a mainstay of her wardrobe;

- Not trendy at all;

- Minimal use of print and pattern; solids in "safe" colors are her go-to's;

- Accessories are understated;

- Hair is well-groomed and not likely to change over time.

The compliment the Traditionalist most likely wants to hear is, "You're so competent and confident."

Examples of Traditionalist style sensibilities include: Hillary Clinton, Laura Bush, Madeleine Albright, Condoleezza Rice and Queen Elizabeth.

The Outdoorsy

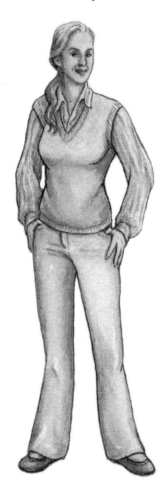

The Outdoorsy woman projects a casual, laid back image, characterized by a friendly, approachable look. It's wholesome, carefree and natural without being sloppy or lazy. Outdoorsy typifies the "all American style" of blue jeans and a button down shirt.

The Outdoorsy woman doesn't think in terms of outfits, but in simple separates that can be mixed and matched easily. Typically, she wears minimal makeup and accessories.

The Outdoorsy woman has a carefree spirit and for her, clothes are a means to an end. She is not trying to be fashionable but functional. She tends to have a very active lifestyle so her closet likely includes a large proportion of sportswear. For work, she keeps it simple.

Her fashion style:

- Casual and relaxed while still having a classic and tailored undertone;

- Mix-and-match separates that are easy to co-ordinate. Use of layering;

- Loosely structured, comfortable shape that covers rather than emphasizes her figure;

- Functional, sportswear designs;

- Jeans are an integral part of her wardrobe as are T-shirts and blazers;

- Hair and makeup are low maintenance;

- Minimal accessories.

The compliment the Outdoorsy most likely wants to hear is, "You're such fun to be with."

Celebrities who best represent the Outdoorsy image are Jane Fonda, Jennifer Aniston, Katherine Hepburn, Lauren Hutton and Natalie Portman.

The Sophisticate

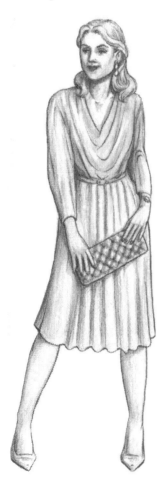

The Sophisticate projects a refined, stately and high maintenance image which is characterized by a cultivated and polished look. Her appearance is impeccably put together from head to toe and her clothes and accessories are worn for status and prestige.

This woman is very elegant and values quality as much as style. She is always well groomed and her look is timeless and streamlined. The Sophisticate will never be caught with her nails "not done" or her hair tousled. She probably does not ever have a reason to wear a T-shirt.

The Sophisticate has a lifestyle that is very much a part of her look. She has a reason to get dressed up for galas, luncheons, board meetings, or cocktails and the resources to invest in the very best quality. She likely has a personal shopper on her team.

Her fashion style:

- Elegant, ensemble dressing where all pieces blend together perfectly;

- Impeccable workmanship, in simple but well-cut proportions, that gently follow her silhouette;

- Minimal details;

- Timeless fashion sensibilities over trendy looks;

- Favors monochromatic tones with no strong contrasts;

- Hair is coiffed to a "T" and makeup is to perfection;

- Accessories are expensive and of the highest quality - lavish even, yet still understated;

- Designer shoes and handbags.

The compliment the Sophisticate most likely wants to hear is, "You have impeccable taste."

Celebrities who embody this style include: Princess Di, Jackie O, Cate Blanchett, and Catherine Deneuve.

The Seductress

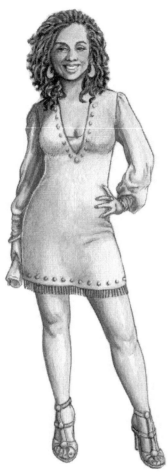

The Seductress projects a sexy and glamorous image which is characterized by a daring and provocative look. Her appearance is sensuous, uninhibited, exciting and designed to reveal and emphasize her feminine silhouette.

Layering is not an option for the Seductress. She likes to show some skin and attract male attention. She selects clothes that flatter her body shape. High-style fashion is secondary.

The Seductress will rarely, if ever, be seen in baggy, loose fitting clothes. If an item does not enhance her sensuality—she is not inclined to wear it. Animal prints are definitely part of her closet, as is sexy lingerie, patterned stockings and stiletto heels.

Her fashion style:

- Non-classical outfits that emphasize body shape with darts often included to slim waist and define bust;

- Tops, skirts and pants designed to hug the body's contours;

- Tapered hems or cutaways to display legs, waist, chest and shoulders;

- She will opt for shorter length dresses and skirts;

- She is very comfortable showing cleavage;

- Her lips will frequently be painted in a shade of red. Her makeup overall is dramatic and seductive (think smoky eyes);

- Her favorite accessories are waist cinching belts, thigh-high boots, dangly earrings, chokers, anklets and toe rings;

- Her hair can be in any style—what is important is that it has movement or looks touchable.

The compliment the Seductress most likely wants to hear is, "You look so sexy."

Celebrities rocking the Seductress style include: Dita Von Teese, Beyonce, Jennifer Lopez, Scarlett Johansson, Sophia Loren, Mariah Carey and Kim Kardashian.

The Romantic

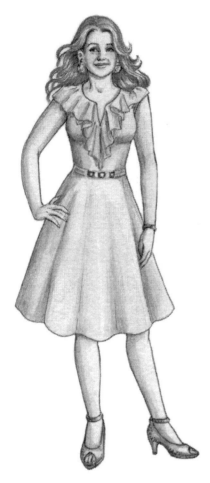

The Romantic woman projects a feminine image characterized by a soft, gentle, and delicate look. Her clothes and accessories are ladylike, dainty, and often worn modestly to cover her body. The Romantic embraces ruffles, bows, lace, long flowing skirts and feminine dresses.

The Romantic woman also tends to be family and home oriented—she may love cooking and entertaining or planning events. She relishes and embraces her femininity and is drawn to designs that express that sensibility. Even her voice may be soft or of a higher pitch quality.

The Romantic will prefer shoes with a dainty look. Her hair will be soft, wavy and on the longer side. Her accessories will be dainty with girly flourishes. She will never be seen in an outfit that has an "edgier" vibe or in clothing that shows too much skin. Yes, she can be sexy, but it will be subtle, not overt.

Her fashion style:

- Soft, gently curved lines that flow loosely over the body;

- Non-structured, more rounded/softer shapes—jackets and coats have natural shoulders;

- Designs will have delicate accents: intricate details such as pintucks, smocking, ruffles, lace, bows, floral appliqués and scalloped edges;

- Bodices and sleeves may be tucked and gathered to add fullness;

- Floral print designs;

- Pretty shoes and makeup;

- Jewelry is definitely part of her ensembles, but delicate rather than statement making;

- Hair is soft, flowing and likely long.

The compliment the Romantic most likely wants to hear is, "You look so pretty tonight."

The Romantic look is embraced by celebrities like: Jane Seymour, Elizabeth Taylor, Penelope Cruz, Eva Longoria Parker and Taylor Swift.

The Eclectic

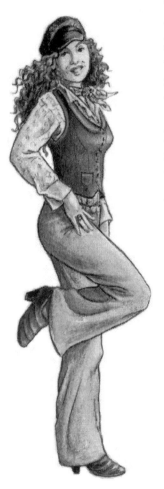

The Eclectic woman projects an original and artistic image which is characterized by a free spirited and independent look. Her appearance is quirky, unconventional, imaginative, and embodies one-of-a-kind dressing, which can make it hard to define. She likes to loudly proclaim her presence with bold fashion choices.

Eclectically styled women are hard to miss, so the message is understood. Clothing and accessories are extreme—either excessive or minimal. Outfits are put together to display and define personality. They thrive on taking fashion risks.

Unlike the Traditionalist, the Eclectic loves mixing things up in her closet and exploring unconventional pairings. She wants to be unique. However, she is not a slave to fashion trends. She likely sets them herself! Her hair and makeup changes with her mood, and her accessories are one of a kind finds.

Her fashion style:

- Radical - like reversing the V in a sweater to the back;

- Bold mixes of pattern, fabric, colors and styles;

- She will shop vintage and consignment to snag unusual finds;

- Statement making accessories are part of her wardrobe arsenal;

- Her clothing is as much an expression of her personality as it is her fashion sense;

- She rarely wears the same ensemble twice;

- She likely has a lot of clothes in her closet;

- Her makeup is used to enhance her outfit de jour;

- Her hair can be very expressive of her fashion sensibility.

The compliment the Eclectic most likely wants to hear is, "You are one of a kind."

Eclectic celebrities include: Sarah Jessica Parker, Diane Keaton, Kate Moss, Whoopie Goldberg, Chloe Sevigny and Gwen Stefani.

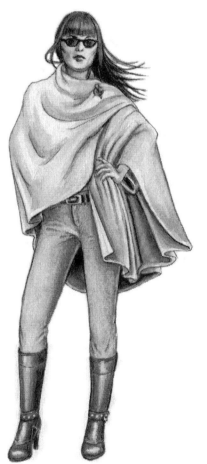

The Diva
The Diva aims to make a fashion-statement which is characterized by striking and exaggerated clothes and accessories. The Diva seeks attention and that "star quality" by being overly dramatic in her choice of cut, silhouette, color or design.

The Diva can be seen with dramatic hats, statement hair styles, and large glasses/sunglasses as signatures. Jackets are also an integral part of her wardrobe, generally with an element of exaggeration—broad shoulders, unusual proportions or extreme lengths.

Bold color choices are definitely par for the course for the Diva, as are dramatic prints and patterns. The Diva is all about standing out, so she will break rules and march by the beat of her own drum just to command attention and create shock value. Unlike the Eclectic, the Diva wants attention for attention's sake. The world is her stage and she uses fashion and style as props. For the woman with Diva style, it's SO all about her.

Her fashion style:

- Sleek, angled or dramatic straight lines;

- Stark, architectural design with emphasis on one feature. She is drawn to edgy designs;

- Contrasts are bright and intense;

- Makeup is vivid and can be over the top;

- Hair is generally part of the Diva package and she will have a signature "do";

- Accessories will be large and statement making;

- Clothing is worn for drama and to make a grand entrance.

The compliment the Diva most likely wants to hear is, "You're such a Diva."

Well known Divas include Lady Gaga, Cher, Grace Jones, Rhianna and Diana Ross.

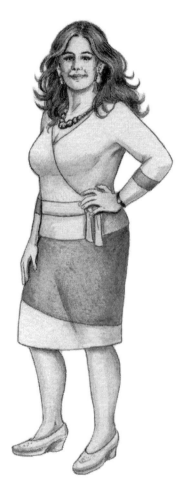

Blended Styles

The seven core styles we just discussed, are foundations for you to use as you begin to develop your own signature. Each style described above is distinct and meant to be the extreme of that sensibility. This is to really drive the point home that each style is comprised of varying factors that may or may not be an *exact* fit for you.

Some women wear their personal style like a comfortable pair of shoes, while others find their style varies according to their mood or environment.

A lot of women I coach, automatically define their style as the Traditionalist because they work in a corporate environment; so their wardrobe staples are tailored suits. But this usually isn't their *signature*. They just don't realize they haven't tapped into *that* yet.

Sometimes a woman, who by default thinks she is Traditionalist, discovers she is more influenced by The Romantic, because the blouses she wears with her corporate suit are in soft pastels with ruffles, and her favorite item of clothing outside of work is a floral, long flowing skirt that softly drapes around her calves that she wears with ballerina flats.

How does she define her style? Well, it's a blend of Traditionalist and Romantic. And what makes it her signature are the ways in which she combines these two styles and makes it her own.

In the same way, I encourage you to be inspired by the 7 core styles to find within them your true signature. Most women are a blend of two or more styles. Create your signature by the unique spin you integrate into your look, so it has your indelible stamp.

"FASHION FADES, STYLE IS ETERNAL"

This famous quote, attributed to Yves St Laurent, really sums up the point of this chapter. Finding your unique style has everything to do with who you are and your self-expression. Your personal style is influenced by so many things least of which should be the fashion de jour. Your lifestyle, ethnicity, culture, experiences, personality, preferences, upbringing and tastes are just a few of the things that dictate whether you lean towards a more classic sensibility or to an edgier one. When examining personal styles, the idea is to think beyond your default style and truly tap into your essence and personality. Sure, your default style may be your style, but I've often found it's usually a combo of several styles for most women. What are you *really* drawn to? What design aesthetics really make you come alive? What would you dare to wear if only you gave yourself permission? What if I told you all it took to Flaunt a particular style was the confidence to do so?

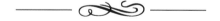

TRANSFORMATION IN ACTION:
MEET SHARON

Sharon is a busy stay-at-home mom with 2 kids. She is 35 years old, of average height and has an ideal figure. Sharon's default uniform was jeans and a shirt. But she started feeling as boring as she looked and wanted a change. Sharon is very pretty: green eyes, light brown shoulder length curly hair and an engaging warm smile. She knew she could do more with her look, and wanted to but she just didn't know quite where to start. After all, she really needed her clothes for the myriad of children's activities she was involved in, the twice a month date night with her hubby, and the occasional meeting with friends. And occasionally, she volunteered at a local school. Essentially, Sharon needed a casual/social wardrobe with "oomph" that reflected her vibrant spirit and made her look as fabulous as she wanted to feel.

When tapping into Sharon's personal style preferences, it became readily apparent that she was a girl's girl. She loved pink, flowers and kittens. Really! She was just oozing Romantic through and through, but her closet reflected a hodge podge of plain shirts, crazy patterns, long drab dresses and the occasional jacket, most which conveyed "I am old and dowdy" instead of "I am young, pretty and alluring and I want to Flaunt It". Sharon's (quick) transformation became easy once we honed in on her style. Pink and other soft but lively hues looked great on her. She loved ruffles, bows, lace and soft drapey fabrics. We added a number of skirts and wrap dresses to her wardrobe, cuter shoes, and a few alluring pieces to help her look like a siren when she was out with her husband. Softly tailored jackets were added so she could mix 'n match with slacks, jeans or skirts when she wanted to project more command. And she started building a collection of really fun accessories to give her ensembles more of an 'edge'.

Sharon made quite the transformation. She soaked up all the advice like a sponge and now is quite the fashionista. Her lifestyle has not changed. She is still a stay-at-home mom. But now, she struts to the PTA meetings in her cute heels, waist cinched with a belt, and is the best dressed mom in her town. More importantly, she looks and feels fabulous because she is now expressing her true essence. What an awesome role model for her daughter.

Observation: *Stay-at-home moms, often by default, believe they are 'outdoorsy' because of their lifestyle spending time with kids; but often when probed, I discover their true style can be far more interesting — it is just lying dormant waiting to be unleashed. A stay-at-home mom can have a signature style that incorporates elements of Outdoorsy, Eclectic and Seductress. In Sharon's case, her style was grounded in Romantic with a touch of Seductress and a dose of Outdoorsy. She just had to get clear, as you will, on what she really liked, the styles she admired, and how she wanted to look and feel in her clothes.*

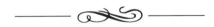

A signature style is distinct. It is an expression of your tastes, personality, goals, lifestyle and more. How do you know when you've found your signature? You feel it and know it on a gut level. When you are rocking your unique look, you'll walk differently, feel amazing and most certainly get compliments.

Somewhere within, you have a unique style trademark; maybe not who you are right now, but who you want to be and want to present to the world. My advice is to experiment. Try adding one or two new elements and see how you feel. If it feels great, then you've got a new style variation. Yay for you! At the end of the day, you have to feel fabulous, whatever your style. Dare to take risks, but always be you.

BE INSPIRED BY FASHION ICONS

Do you have a fashion icon or someone whose style inspires you? The answer is typically very revealing because it helps crystallize your style aspirations. And often, that fashion icon's style is a reflection of your ideal signature style.

Your particular fashion inspiration doesn't necessarily have to be a celebrity; it can be any woman whose style you admire and would love to make yours. But in most cases a celebrity comes to mind more readily because they are featured everywhere we look.

Let's look at celebrities who possess a signature style that is so distinctive and inspirational they are all considered to be fashion icons in their own right:

- **The Duchess of Cambridge, Kate Middleton,** has emerged as a style icon that women the world over aspire to emulate. And it is no surprise. She has an impeccable sense of chic that is sophisticated and classic yet still absolutely relatable. She Flaunts a fabulous blend of Sophisticate meets Romantic, anchored in Traditionalist sensibilities.

- **Audrey Hepburn**. Audrey, the quintessential Sophisticate, is considered to be the queen of classic elegance and chic sophistication. She is still the gold standard against whom all newcomers are judged.

- **Josephine Baker**. Josephine was a 'Diva' decades ahead of her time, who took fashion risks and bucked the system to make an indelible mark in fashion history.

- **Marilyn Monroe.** Who played the Seductress better than Marilyn? She oozed coquettish sex appeal and allure. Newcomer Sofia Vergara is re-inventing Marilyn's sexy style with 21st century attitude. Her personal brand hinges on Flaunting her killer curves.

- **Michelle Obama.** Michelle is a fashion icon that truly has an accessible style. She defines Traditionalist with a dash of panache. Michelle embraces color and loves clean silhouettes, like the sheath dress. She is poised and elegant. And she accessorizes marvelously to make traditional looks her own. Traditionalist yes, but also Sophisticate and Romantic.

- **Natalie Portman.** Natalie has an easy, breezy style that enhances her amazing figure and petite stature. She always looks comfortable and understated, classic but never uptight, pretty but never overdone. A fine example of Outdoorsy meets Traditionalist meets Romantic.

- **Sarah Jessica Parker.** Sarah is an example of a woman who is not afraid to take risks. She is very fashion forward, trendy, and likes to mix things up for creative edge while still remaining feminine. She is a grounded in Eclectic with a healthy dose of Romantic.

- **Angelina Jolie.** Angelina is an example of a woman who blends her signature styles. When she is in mommy mode, she tends to stick to neutral tones and clean lines; but when she dresses up, she favors understated colors, simple silhouettes and elegant styling. And those eyes and lips. If that's not alluring I don't know what is! But at her core, Angelina is a mix of Traditionlist and Sophisticate.

- **Jennifer Aniston.** Jennifer epitomizes casual, effortless style. She is usually seen in a great fitting pair of jeans and a simple classic shirt under a blazer, with perhaps a scarf as an accent. Her accessories and makeup are very understated and her signature hair is a straight blow out, but always picture perfect. Outdoorsy with a dab of Traditionalist defines her look.

- **Queen Latifah.** The Queen is a lady who embraces her body with such confidence, that you don't notice what size she is. She always dresses appropriately for the occasion, whether in a gown or more laid back sporty separates. Her style sensibilities lean heavily toward Outdoorsy's.

- **Beyonce**. With Beyonce you get drama, glamour and definite sex appeal, all in one package. She is not afraid of her curves and loves to Flaunt them in figure hugging silhouettes. Beyonce is a blend of Seductress and Diva, no question.

- **Victoria Beckham**. Victoria is the ultimate fashionista who embraces dramatic, edgy styling with her signature designer handbags, huge sunglasses and wicked heels. Sophisticate meets Diva!

- **Lady Gaga.** A Diva to the nth degree. Everything Lady Gaga wears is about getting attention. She takes her hair, makeup, accessories, and clothing to extremes. She lives for shock value.

- **Nicole Richie.** Nicole has really emerged as a fashion aficionado who really embodies an Eclectic style. She expresses this in an easy breezy bohemian sensibility with her love of head ties, print and maxi dresses.

- **Coco Chanel**. The one and only. She dared to embrace her masculine side and it was this that made her designs (and their fabrication) so unique in their time. She spoke her mind and did not care what people thought. This takes guts. The same guts it took to wear her lovers' trousers and jackets and style them to suit her tastes. Seductress? Sure. Eclectic? Absolutely. Diva? Darn right.

FLAUNT YOUR SIGNATURE STYLE

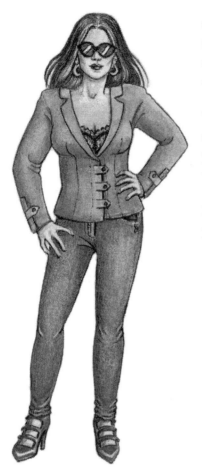

Once you feel comfortable about a particular style that embodies who you are, this becomes the foundation for you to start really having fun with your ensembles.

Work on defining your image based on the personal style that best fits you. And certainly give yourself permission to play with that look to express your unique flair and individuality.

Let's look at some of the ways you can define your personal style and make it your signature:

❖ Do you have something distinctive about your appearance? In my case, it's my 6' frame. It could be the show stopping lips that celebrities like Scarlett Johansson and Angelina Jolie have made famous, or jewel colored eyes like Elizabeth Taylor, or famous legs like Tina Turner, who at 65+ can still rock it out. Perhaps you can make a body attribute part of your signature look.

❖ Utilize a signature accessory. One of my clients uses scarves in a variety of colors, patterns and shapes and wears them with all her suits to spice up her look. Celebrities who have developed famous trademarks include Victoria Beckham and her signature handbags and sunglasses, Halle Berry's pixie, Sarah Palin's glasses, Rihanna's ever changing edgy hair and Beyonce's oversized earrings. Meryl Streep's character in "The Devil Wears Prada" was always adorned with a white Hermes scarf, whether as part of her outfit or used as an accessory. Find your equivalent.

❖ Refine your personal style and make it yours; whether you tend to gravitate towards monochromatic silhouettes with a complementary splash of color in your shoes, or like to create an edgy mix of dramatic accessories you use in new and surprising ways. You will find that you will tweak and further refine your signature style, as you become more comfortable with what flatters you and as you step outside your "safe" zone. Learn to experiment and be bold with your choices to fully realize your style potential.

❖ Is there something unconventional about you? A different accent? An unusual feature? Cindy Crawford's mole has made her look distinctive, while Barbra Streisand has made her profile famous with her less-than-perfect nose. Singer Mary J. Blige has made the scar under her left eye which has become her trademark beauty mark—she doesn't try to cover it up. It makes her unique. All these women have transformed a negative facial feature into their signature look and worked it to the max. Any attribute that is unique to you can be artfully used to reinforce your signature.

Like anything that's worth it, developing your signature style won't happen overnight; but it will happen with time, effort, dedication and enthusiasm. It's exciting and empowering to build an image progressively that is in sync with your character and personality. It's all about packaging your signature look so that everything is in alignment.

I know that it can feel scary and take you way out of your comfort zone. But the question you have to ask yourself is: What is the worst thing that can happen?

Let's say, you take a risk and try on an outfit that you like, but it doesn't work for you. If you didn't try it on, you would never know whether it was going to look "wow" or "whoa" on you. And maybe you surprise yourself and that outfit you try looks sensational. It's not like anything you currently have in your wardrobe and it works. That's a wonderful experience!

That's what refining your signature style is all about: experimenting, taking calculated fashion risks and being inspired to try different looks so that eventually nailing your signature style becomes second nature. The key is knowing what styles to look for, how to pair items with each other so they work in harmony and how to pull together your ensembles so that they express you.

Over time (or with professional assistance), you will learn the skills to instinctively know what works for you. Your eye will become trained to see the potential in clothing and visualize an item paired with others you own and accented with accessories. You will gain the confidence to try new looks that you believe are in sync with your sensibilities. And, you will be inspired by women you admire and take pieces of their style trademarks and rework them to suit you.

Over time, we all grow, change and evolve and so it is with your style; it needs to evolve alongside you. Your signature style is not static. As your lifestyle changes, your needs and goals change; and perhaps your circumstances, career and aspirations change, hence your signature style will morph into something new and wonderful as well.

Just as you need to embrace the changes in your life, be willing and prepared to embrace the changes that will undoubtedly occur in your personal style, so that it continues to reflect the woman you are. Be brave and allow your ever-increasing knowledge, self-assuredness and confidence to radiate through your unique signature, effortless style.

BECOMING FABULOUS

Go back to the 7 positive adjectives you wrote down in Chapter 1 that describe the person you are or how you would like to be perceived by others. And then, consider those attributes and how they can best be reflected in your signature style.

For example, if you would like to be perceived as confident, how can you express confidence in your personal style? Perhaps you wear bold colors like tomato red, violet, or cobalt blue, if these hues work on you. Perhaps you look for blazers with strong shoulders to convey more presence. Perhaps it is as subtle as the way you stand and walk. Perhaps it's because you dare to wear things in unconventional ways, such as a dress as a tunic. The options are as endless as your imagination allows.

I encourage my clients to keep a scrapbook so they can continually redefine and update their style, by collecting pictures from magazines, catalogues and websites that reflect their preferred look.

Make that your homework from this chapter. Find your inspiration from within and from the women around you or those in magazines. Just look at what you are drawn to and don't worry too much about cost, lifestyle or your body type. The goal is to start to see the patterns in what you like and to start to incorporate these patterns in ways that work for your body, lifestyle and goals. It doesn't take a fortune to look fabulous. Just know how.

Chapter Six
Your Wardrobe's 'Backbone'

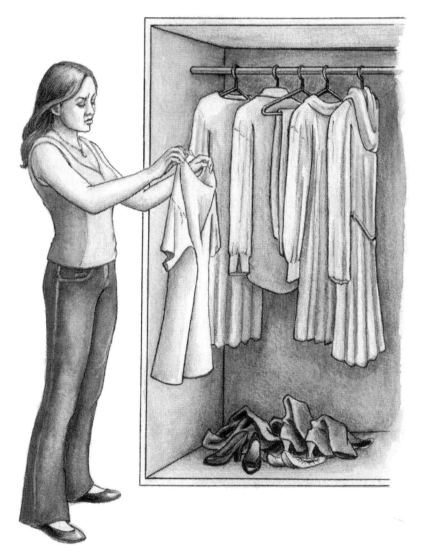

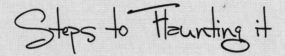

Steps to Flaunting it

✦ Having a wardrobe with a backbone means having all your bases covered, with a range of flattering basics that form the foundations from which you can build a stunning closet of pieces that can be mixed and matched.

✦ Many of these key wardrobe basics require multiples. You need a variety of styles of dresses, skirts, pants, tops and jackets to have a truly versatile wardrobe.

✦ Start creating a wardrobe you love. Stop adding clothes to your closet, "just because". Your new mission is to add clothes that perfectly compliment you and help reinforce the messages you want to convey via your appearance.

✦ Take the time and effort to discover items which mirror your signature style. Your wardrobe should delight and inspire you.

✦ Always choose pieces that feel comfortable and make you feel fabulous. If you feel fabulous, you'll look fabulous!

IN THE CLOSET

There is so much you can learn from a woman by looking at her closet. When you think about it, the closet is a reflection of the woman herself - her lifestyle, preferences, favorite colors, fashion sensibility, and personal style (or lack thereof). If I were to look in your closet right now what would it say about you? Are you liking its message?

A closet is so much more than the clothes in it. It's not supposed to be a hodge podge of items, carelessly hung in the same compartment with no rhyme or reason for how those items got there. There is a reason you bought that lime green suit after all, whether it looks amazing or awful on you. Do you believe you are more fabulous than your wardrobe? Then, ask yourself why your clothes don't reflect the gem you are. Better yet, consider when you go shopping, who you are shopping for; the woman you are, the women you wish you were, or the woman you used to be?

Think of your wardrobe as you would your very own clothing "collection". Imagine multiple versions of you walking down a runway in your clothes. Are you hiding your eyes or brimming with pride? Gotcha there, didn't I?

One of the reasons so many women dread getting dressed every day is because their closet does not reflect them or who they aspire to be. They are frustrated because they have a vision of how they want to be perceived in their mind's eye, however vague, and yet their wardrobe does not have the pieces to bring this vision to reality. So the woman ends up complaining about her clothes or that she has nothing to wear. In truth, often the real issue is that she does not have a closet full of pieces she loves, that work together to help her create the looks of her choosing. Her wardrobe does not have a "soul"—HER soul.

There are so many emotional associations we have with our clothes, least of which may be whether they even suit us at all. So often we buy something for the wrong reasons: because we need an outfit for an occasion; because it's on sale; because our friend /sister/ mother/ loved one told us to buy it; because it's safe; it's comfortable; it looked so cute on the hanger....and so on.

Ladies, these aren't the reasons to buy clothing. You buy a piece of clothing because it suits your body, it fits you, it's in synch with your style, it is the right color for you, it can work with other pieces in your closet, it looks fabulous on you, and most importantly because you love it.

Let me make the wardrobe conundrum a littler simpler for you.

There are specific items of clothing that make up the backbone of every closet. Without these core pieces, it is challenging, at best, to really make your wardrobe work for you. Each item has a specific role to play and once you have a handle on what those essential items are and how to wear them with pizzazz, clothes shopping will become easier and you will start creating a wardrobe you love.

You may already own some of these key pieces in one form or another. My goal in this chapter is help you understand why these items are your wardrobe's backbone and to share tips on how to wear each for maximum impact.

So let's look at what I deem to be the **13 Key Pieces of a Woman's Wardrobe** and how you can mix, match and integrate these core pieces with each other so you create effortlessly pulled together looks repeatedly. Are you ready?

1) THE WHITE SHIRT

No woman can have too many white shirts. They are the classic wardrobe staple.

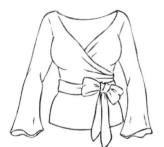

White shirts came out of the closet (so to speak) when Sharon Stone wore a simple white Gap shirt (it was her husband's at the time) to the Oscars many years ago, that she tucked and tied in the back with a voluminous satin skirt. She took that basic and made it high fashion. And she looked unbelievably stunning in her ensemble.

But wait. Let's get clear now. *White shirt* does not mean your husband's/boyfriend's/father's boxy, plain white shirt. Sharon is an exception because she wore a man's shirt creatively. When I urge you to add white shirts to your closet, I'm talking about fitted, feminine-enhanced white shirts, that are designed for a woman's silhouette. Ruffled, corseted, zipped, cuffed, ruched, contoured, you name it; there are many options awaiting your selection. The style of shirt you choose has to suit your personal style, figure, and the occasion, which is why multiples are a must.

A white shirt with a touch of stretch will take you from day to night with ease (and without wrinkles!) It's like working on a blank canvas, so you can quickly glam it up for evening excitement with statement accessories, or tone it down for more casual affairs.

How to Wear Your White Shirt

❖ Nothing says style quite like a classic white shirt and the perfect pair of tailored blue jeans or black pants and cute heels. Pair with a blazer worn open and voila! You have re-created Jennifer Aniston's "uniform". This combination works because it is timeless and effortless.

❖ If you are pear-shaped or disguising a large tummy, choose a tailored shirt that sits a couple of inches below your waist—it can camouflage a multitude of sins. The latest corset-style shirts help minimize large waists, as do shirts with ruching at the sides.

❖ If white isn't so right on you, add a pop of color with a bold necklace in turquoise, coral, jet-black or bamboo; or add a scarf, cardigan or jacket in one of your signature colors.

❖ And always buy a shirt in the right size so there is no gaping around the button holes. Don't forget what you learned about fit.

An important point:
You might be wondering why I specified "white". A white shirt is the most versatile colored shirt to own. It is the **fastest path to effortless** for shirts. No other colored shirt is quite as crisp, clean or classic. But I do not want you to think that you should only have white shirts in your closet! By all means DO add shirts in your "wow" colors to your collection as well. In fact, I highly recommend it.

2) A PERFECT FITTING PAIR OF JEANS

More than 20 years ago, a young Brooke Shields shimmied into a pair of skin-tight Calvin Klein jeans, with a partially unbuttoned white shirt, and gushed on TV screens across the world, *"Nothing comes between me and my Calvins."*

That ad campaign made its mark in advertising history, but also firmly established the denim blue jean as a wardrobe staple. Let's face it, jeans aren't going away any time soon. In fact, every year designers make radical improvements in fit, design and fabric that make them an indispensable part of a woman's wardrobe.

In today's culture, at least one fabulous pair of jeans is an *essential* essential, and like the classic white shirt, you can dress jeans up or down. Jeans can take you from casual to social and back again just by pairing them with different tops and accessories. Because of the versatility and effortless nature of dressing with jeans as your foundation, finding a pair that fit as though they were personally tailored just for you is a top priority.

To help take some of the mystery out of figuring out why certain jeans fit you better than others, here are some key pointers.

7 Keys TO FINDING THE PERFECT FITTING JEANS

1. There are many styles and cuts of jeans. Understanding the basics will help you find a flattering cut.

    o   **Boot cut jeans** work for most women, especially those who are triangular shaped or round. The flared lower leg balances wide hips and thighs.

    o   **Trouser style jeans** work for triangle and plus-sized figures and those who prefer more room in the thigh.

    o   Who can wear **skinny jeans**? As the name implies, this style is best suited for women who are slim through the thighs, hips and bottom, especially slim inverted triangles and rectangles. The skinny jean is meant to fit tight all the way down the leg, so they look great when paired with a tunic top or mini dress.

    o   **Straight leg** jeans are the epitome of the classic American relaxed style blue jeans and a white Tee, *a la* Cindy Crawford relaxing in the Bahamas. Straight legs are universally flattering, especially on inverted triangles and rectangular shapes.

    o   **Boyfriend** style jeans work with most figure shapes and have a more casual vibe. They tend to be very roomy in the thigh and cuffed. Round figures should avoid this cut as it may make you appear larger.

o The latest **curvy cut** jeans are great for those with fuller hips, thighs and bottoms. They look amazing on an hourglass as well as triangle figures because they accommodate and flatter curves.

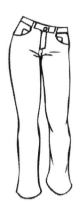

2. To **stretch** or not to stretch? Quite frankly, ever since designers started adding spandex to jeans, I have never looked back. The stretch enables jeans to hug you in all the right places without the binding you feel from the non-stretch variety. The spandex allows the jeans to follow the contours of a woman's body and ultimately makes her curves look that much more shapely. Additionally, stretch in the fabric allows jeans to rebound better after multiple wearings, unlike the non-stretch styles that literally get stretched totally out of shape. My advice? Look for 2% spandex in the fabric and you can't go wrong.

3. **Back pockets** are important because, depending on how big, long and far apart they are, they can drastically change the way you look from behind. If you have a small tush, look for jeans with back pockets that are widely spaced. They will add more shape to your bottom. Same goes for pockets with flaps. They add bulk at the rear. Avoid overly big pockets because they can make you look as if you have no tush at all.

   If you have a cushy tush, go for the opposite. Avoid pockets with flaps or ornate designs as they will draw attention to your rear end. Look for decent sized pockets that sit right on the highest point of your bottom and closer to the waistband. If the pockets are too small, they will make you look larger from the back, and if they are too far down, they will make you look as though your rear goes on forever.

4. A variety of **washes** are now available, particularly in almost bleached-out blue-white, gray wash and blue/black tones. Very faded jeans are not as popular now as they were in the 90's. A medium blue wash is great for a casual look, while a darker wash is suitable for more dressed up occasions.

   Darker washes, from dark blue to dark gray and all the way to black are more versatile in general, because they can be dressed up or down and convey a more polished look. These shades can be the best choice for women with full hips or thighs as the darker colors camouflage.

5. In and out of style are very **distressed jeans**, whether shredded, torn, thrashed or otherwise basically ruined. Personally, for the over 35 crowd I don't think this look is the most age appropriate choice. However, if your personal style is very edgy/rocker vibe or creative, and this look really appeals to you, you should follow your instincts.

6. **Say "no" to** 1) overly ornate designs (flowers, embroidery, glitter and studs—the 70s are over, girlfriend!), 2) dirty or stone washes, as they look sloppy, 3) whisker wash embellishments as they are typically not flattering and 4) super low rises suitable for thinner teenage girls. And of course, any jeans that don't fit properly or flatter and enhance your curves!

7. **Brands to test drive.** A brand of jeans quite a few of my clients love is **NYDJ** (Not Your Daughter's Jeans). The company's mission is to allow women to feel good in their jeans in the bodies they have now. My philosophy exactly! Built with their proprietary "Lift/Tuck" technology, the jean tucks tummies and lifts and supports the rear. I can attest to this because I have seen it do so on many bodies. It also has one of the highest rises you're likely to find in a jean, (11" in the front and even higher in the rear), so they really flatter women who have "womanly" bodies. The higher rise makes for a more comfortable fit in the crotch and minimizes "muffin tops" and "butt peekaboos" (Amen!). There is also considerable stretch throughout which makes for a jean that really contours to your body. Because the jean lifts and tucks, you will look smaller wearing them (Do I hear another Amen?). If you are a curvy girl, it may be worth trying a pair. This jean has liberated the wardrobes (and self-esteem) of many "curvy" women.

My favorite pair of jeans that fits my body exceptionally is **CJ** by Cookie Johnson. Finally a jean with a generous 34" inseam that I can buy in the store that looks bootylicious too! Having had the pleasure of meeting Cookie Johnson herself when she launched the jeans at Nordstrom Tysons in Virginia in 2009, I applaud her mission as well (I am paraphrasing from our brief interview)—to offer curvy women options in different styles which are all cut fuller in the hips, thigh and rear, which are equipped with contoured waistbands, in a lighter weight denim fabric that feels so comfortable on the body. The jeans are sewn and embroidered with finesse on the outside—no huge logos on your tush—with her signature red lining on the inside, so soft you don't even feel like you're wearing jeans. You'll get comfort, great fit, and style, in a wide range of sizes from these jeans.

Now after reading these tips, I don't want to hear complaints about not finding the perfect pair of jeans. Yes, there are tons of styles, brands and cuts; and it can be overwhelming. And yes, you're going to have to try many pairs on before finding your true style. But I promise you, when you find that perfect pair, it will be so worth it. Another **fastest path to effortless** is having a couple of GREAT fitting jeans in your closet.

3) BLACK DRESS PANTS

Every woman needs at least one pair (if not more) of classic black slacks in her wardrobe because they are simply so versatile, elegant and figure flattering. Every color matches black. You can pair a variety of tops, jackets, shirts and cardigans with black pants. Plus, black is the ultimate slimming hue. There are few closets that don't have this basic.

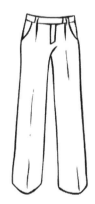

But, like jeans, finding the perfect pair of black slacks that fit you in all the right places can be challenging. However, it's the one wardrobe basic I encourage you to work extra hard at. Exquisitely tailored black trousers define and silhouette your body's shape and move with you to enhance your look, whether you're sitting, standing, or (heaven forbid), bending over. The look is easy, classic and effortless.

Conversely, a pair of ill-fitting trousers greatly diminishes how pulled together you look. Pulling at the seams, gaping at the closure, puddles of fabric near the crotch or wrinkling there, are all image deal breakers. Take the time to search out brands and invest in a quality pair that is perfectly cut for your body shape—they are out there, I promise you.

Classic black pants can last season after season, so it pays to do the math. If you own a pair of superbly crafted Calvin Klein's you paid $200 for and wear them 50 times, isn't that a better deal than the brand you bought at the local store for $30 that you wore once or twice? Believe me, the investment in quality is worth it in the long run.

Like every item in your wardrobe, ensure the fit is right for your body shape. Review the section on your figure type for suggestions on the type of slacks that best flatter you.

Of course, it also goes without saying that the top, shirt or jacket you wear with your black pants is integral to how stylish your ensemble looks. Whether you pair your slacks with a pretty blouse, blazer, or tunic top, be sure you pay attention to the proportions in your ensemble for maximum appeal.

TRANSFORMATION IN ACTION:
MEET ALEX

Alex is a busy entrepreneur who needs to project a strong personal brand for her business. She has a wonderful figure at 38, but she needed help with her wardrobe. When I diagnosed Alex's closet, what became glaringly obvious was that she was missing many key essential pieces—critical aspects of her wardrobe's "backbone". Alex was by no means a fashionista, but what was really interesting about her closet was that she had invested in some really unique pieces, especially jackets and sweaters. I was excited by some of these items and saw how they meshed well with her creative/sporty style sense. The items on their own were really fabulous. The problem, however, was that she did not have the right complementary pieces to pair with these amazing tops.

For example, Alex owned this really cool black zippered jacket but did not own a bottom that would enable her to Flaunt It. So the jacket hung in her closet, unworn. She had many items like this—items she bought because of their uniqueness and style that did not go with the pieces she already owned to create ensembles. To make matters worse, Alex's closet was one of the leanest I've seen. She really didn't own many clothes, far less accessories like jewelry, handbags and shoes. Here we had a closet with a few amazing pieces but with no mates and lacking core pieces, period. It was no wonder Alex could never find anything to wear!

My work with Alex largely involved creating a shopping list for her so she could start filling in the gaps in her closet (slacks, perfect jeans, underpinnings, shoes etc.). And importantly, ensuring she had the right partners to wear with her amazing jackets and sweaters. She had a defined style sensibility, but it needed focus and augmenting before she could express how fabulous she could look. Once she got her wardrobe's backbone intact, she could begin to wear her unique power jackets and project the command, confidence and assertiveness she needed for her business.

Observation: Alex's wardrobe challenge is not unique, though maybe a tad extreme. Many closets suffer the same fate and for that reason women have difficulty creating outfits from their closets. Without the backbone pieces and accents to complement them, you really don't have a wardrobe. You have an incomplete collection of clothes. Resist the urge to buy the latest trends every season and consider the following:

a) *Do I really need this piece?*

b) *Does this take my image in the right direction?*

c) *Do I own other pieces that I can pair with this?*

d) *Can I get many varied wearings out of this item?*

e) *Will it help make me look fabulous?*

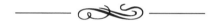

4) THE COCKTAIL DRESS

What woman could say her wardrobe was complete without the essential little cocktail number? The cocktail dress is a classic wardrobe staple and has come to epitomize all that is elegant, sophisticated and alluring about a woman.

A cocktail dress is defined as any dress suited for more formal outings that falls anywhere from just above the knee to ballerina length, (which is just short of the ankle).

In recent years, fashion trends have moved way beyond the "basic black and pearls" statement dressing that fashion icons like Audrey Hepburn personified in the 1950s, to incorporate a rainbow bright palette of colors including scarlet, emerald green, turquoise, fuchsia or any of the multitude of hues that best suit you.

Cocktail dresses incorporate as many styles and varieties as designers can create. In fabrics ranging from floaty organza and chiffon to fine silk, satin, crepe, lace, taffeta or French linen, they present you with the opportunity to let your creative and stylish flair go wild.

The Little Black Dress or the Little Bold Dress?

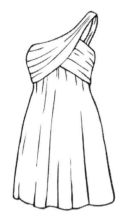

Coco Chanel introduced the little black dress (LBD) in 1926, and over 75 years later its chic simplicity still rules the cocktail hour, making it a style that transcends all that has transpired since its conception.

While it's almost impossible to go wrong with the classic LBD, it has become such a fashion staple that you can often find yourself lost in a sea of little black dresses at social/formal functions.

Besides, black is not a color that suits everyone; so while it may be the easiest and most recognizable solution for after-5 wear, it's not necessarily going to say ooh-la-la for you. And, do you really want to be just another woman in a little black dress among a hundred other women in little black dresses? Do you want to blend into the background, or glimmer like the bright shining star you are, hmmm?

Evening wear is usually about a celebration. How better to celebrate and show your sense of personal style to the world than in a stunning *colored* cocktail dress?

Cocktail dresses can be one of the most fun essential items in your wardrobe. Go ahead and dare to be that Diva you've buried deep inside. The general trend in formal wear is solid blocks of color rather than patterns; so if you're going to wear a color, why not choose one that grabs attention and says boldly, "This is who I am!"?

Forget all the advice you hear and read about the particular colors that are all the rage this season. The designers who dictate fashion trends constantly change the color palettes merely because they can (and because all the slaves to fashion will rush out to buy their latest creations in the latest colors—it's all about clever marketing). Choose your colors based on what makes you look and feel beautiful.

So whether you're rocking your LBD, or its alternative, a 'little bold dress' in your favorite color, let's take a look at how to hook the cocktail dress and reel in as many big fish as you can handle!

HOOK THE COCKTAIL DRESS:
6 Effortless Tips

1. Choose a style that enhances your shape by adding curves where you want them and creating a gorgeous silhouette. Curve enhancers? A deep 'V' neckline which creates a focal point at the waist, making it look smaller. Ruching is also a great curve inducer whether at the waist or sides of a dress. And of course, a belt, sash or waistband at the waist creates curves.

2. Add a touch of bling with eye-popping sparkly earrings, necklace or bracelets (but not all three if you are going for understated elegance).

3. The days of color matching your handbag and shoes with your outfit are well and truly over; so *up the ante* with a silver or gold purse, or go all out with a vibrant color. Nude/skin tone colored shoes are all the rage and I love this look. Make your legs go on forever in a nude or metallic pump for optimal impact.

4. Look for glam embellishments that set your dress apart from the rest and add that 'wow' factor. Lace inserts, sheer panels, beads, bows or ruffles all add to the personality of the dress.

5. What is your style sensibility? Lace, flounces and bows in paler shades suggest femininity and romance, while sharp, minimalist styles suggest trend-setting, effortless style. Gun metal gray, black and deep maroon suggest sophistication and elegance, while vivid colors and unusual shapes say cutting-edge creativity and élan.

6. Gold and silver offer a range of tones that can lift your energy and elegance levels into the stratosphere. If a solid base of either of these colors in your cocktail dress is too much for you, then try a bold stroke with sequins or beads, or add distinctive touches of jewelry to enliven your look and add sparkle.

5) THE JACKET

Like most of the wardrobe staples listed in this chapter, it's highly likely you already have 3 or 4 jackets tucked away in your wardrobe. Therefore, what we are going to discuss is what it takes to transform your basic jacket into one that you'll barely recognize and how to find the perfect jacket for your size and proportions.

Whether you're a stay-at-home mom who wants to add a jacket to her casual jeans and Tee look when she collects the kids from school, or a corporate exec who wants a sleek, sophisticated and stylish number to command attention at the monthly board meeting, your jacket should give you true presence.

The fit must be impeccable, so stick with what works for your body shape and proportions. I typically recommend women wear their jackets buttoned to show off their silhouettes and curves, unless the jacket is meant to be worn open. Too many women wear their jackets or blazers unbuttoned, so the sides flap around sloppily. They lose their contours, wind up looking boxy, and the overall look is less than becoming.

My wish for every woman is that she is proud to show off the curve of her waist, the line of her shoulders or the length of her torso, by wearing a jacket that enhances her body shape.

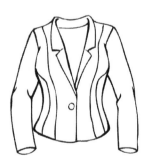

A recent trend I'm loving is ¾ length sleeves, which make your legs look longer—you'll just have to believe me on that one. They are also excellent for women with long arms who can seldom find a suitable sleeve length.

Remember that when you are wearing a jacket, it is the first thing people you meet are going to notice, so ensure your jacket is an investment piece. A sloppy, ill-fitting, badly made jacket is going to send out negative cues instantly, which are going to make you feel bad about yourself and make others think poorly of you.

Think about it: aren't you worth the extra $100 or so dollars for a jacket that makes you look and feel like a *million dollars*?

Let's have a look at ways to nail your jacket essentials.

❖ Like most wardrobe staples we've already discussed, darker shades are more flattering and practical. But that doesn't necessarily mean you have to immediately head to the black, grey and khaki jacket section in the stores. A variety of colors can be equally flattering and practical depending on your color palette.

❖ Tweed fabrics can be a great way to make a classic jacket style more interesting. Hounds-tooth, glen plaid, checks, etc. are all classic patterns that can add subtle color variations, especially in professional settings.

❖ Jacket styles run the gamut from the peplum (which we've discussed), double breasted, military styled, corseted, asymmetrical, wrap, boyfriend, etc. There are many options. What takes you to the fab lane depends on how it flatters you, the occasion, and whether it reinforces your personal style.

❖ For extra pizzazz, experiment with jackets in prints or patterns. This is a great option for Eclectics or Divas who want to be different and to stand out.

6) MUST HAVE UNDERGARMENTS

Every item of clothing in your wardrobe is only going to look as good as the undergarments you wear that give you the proper foundation.

Bras
It's surprising how many women underestimate the power of a well-fitted bra. Did you know that wearing the right bra can:

• take off 10 pounds;

• make you look younger;

• improve your posture;

• show off your waist and torso; and

• support your breasts without discomfort.

Getting proper support from your bra is essential to looking and feeling great. An ill-fitting bra negatively impacts your appearance in the same way ill fitting clothes do. One of my favorite brands for full-figured women, is the Le Mystere bra. Women trying this bra for the first time are often amazed at how their torsos are elongated and how their busts are comfortably supported, so they are in their proper perky position. They see how much better they look in their clothes just by changing their bra.

The fastest path to effortless transformation—wearing the right bra in the right size.

The main points to remember when shopping for the right bra are:

- First get properly fitted! Most women are wearing the wrong size to begin with. Visit your local lingerie boutique (these typically are not the chain store variety) to get an expert to fit you in the right size and style;

- Always buy your bra so that it fits on the loosest clasps—this gives you longer usage because bras slacken with age and you can tighten the clasps as this occurs;

- Nude/skin tone is the most versatile bra color, especially for wearing under white tops. Never wear white under white, although dark skinned women can get away with wearing black under white;

- Never put your bra in the dryer. This destroys the elasticity and drastically shortens your bra's life;

- Your body changes over time so make sure you adjust your foundation garments routinely to accommodate changes.

A good fitting bra should not:

- Feel too loose or too tight across the torso;

- Leave strap marks;

- Create 'boob bubbles' (breasts overflow because bra cup size is too small);

- Create 'headlights' (nipples poking through);

- Ride up in the back (indicates the bra band is too loose); and

- Show bulges of flesh on back of band (indicates the bra band is too tight).

Look for these signs of a good fitting bra:

- Breasts that are at the center of the torso—uplifted and perky;

- The band of the bra is level across your back;

- When you lift your arms, your breasts stay in place;

- Your breasts look symmetrical;

- Your breasts have better definition in your clothes;

- The bra has a smooth finish under your clothes; and

- The bra is comfortable.

Get all these factors right, and you'll be astonished at the difference a good bra can make to your overall image.

Shapewear

Have you ever wondered why celebrities always look so slim and svelte, even in the most figure-hugging outfit imaginable?

Chances are they are using shapewear to give them that lean, streamlined look. Hello Spanx!

Unlike the constricting girdles and corsets of days gone by, today's shapewear is designed to comfortably tuck away unwanted bulges in the tummy, hips, thighs, back or rear (without making you feel like you can't breathe) and making you look fabulous.

The modern materials used in today's shapewear mean that you can look 10 pounds lighter, trimmer, toned and terrific without feeling as if you're enclosed in a steel vice. What's more, the fabric can breathe, so you won't end up feeling as though you're in a soggy wetsuit.

Invest in pieces that smooth unwanted bulges, lift breasts, support your tush or minimize your tummy. Or use them to enhance. Push-up or padded bras and panties are a wonderful way to augment for the less well endowed. Many women can benefit from a little tweaking or refining, can't they?

Shapewear is a woman's secret best friend in the closet, but shhhh! Don't tell anyone.

Pantyhose

A question I'm frequently asked about is pantyhose; whether they should be worn, and if so, what colors are best.

To wear or not to wear? In conservative environments like Government, banking or very corporate cultures, pantyhose is probably a requirement, particularly if you are a senior executive (or aiming to be one). In other professional environments where strict dress codes are not enforced, it really comes down to personal preference.

Let's look at some of the benefits of wearing pantyhose:

- They can provide an extra layer of protective warmth during the colder months;

- They even out skin discolorations and camouflage spider veins and other blemishes;

- They create a smoother line; so dresses, skirts and pants drape more evenly on the body;

- They convey a more formal and conservative look.

But given these benefits, there are also plenty of reasons to forego pantyhose. These include:

- They can be an uncomfortable extra layer during the warmer months;

- Wearing pantyhose is high maintenance because they snag easily;

- Pantyhose are a challenge when wearing sandals (look for the toeless variety if you have to wear stockings with peep toe pumps).

So, my advice is to do whatever makes you feel good. Never mind what your mom told you about what "good girls" do. Exercise your power to choose.

7) THE DAY DRESS

Every woman needs at least one chic, stylish, summery dress in her wardrobe. Yes... even those women who spend their lifetime in jeans will eventually find there comes a time when a dress is required. Why? Because when it's warm outside, a day dress is the ultimate in effortless dressing.

The fastest path to effortless: You find that perfect dress and you're pretty much done clothing wise! Just pair with your favorite sandals or sling backs, add an accessory or two and you have a pulled together, easy breezy look. No worries about what to mix and match with what. And for many women, finding a dress that fits well is simpler than the hunt for the right slacks.

Get on the day dress bandwagon if you're looking for effortless ways to look fabulous. After all, isn't that why you are reading this book?

The variety of shapes, styles, fabrics, textures and colors that could be considered fashionable is virtually limitless; so when searching for the perfect day dress, have an open mind and trust your instincts.

What do I mean? Go with your heart when it comes to overall appeal and personality, but go with your head (and all the advice in this book) to choose the shapes and colors that are designed to suit your silhouette and give you that "ka-pow" factor we've been mentioning.

Let's look at a few design elements that you want to consider when looking for casual dresses:

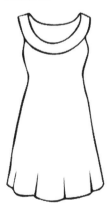

❖ Details including peep holes, sleeve length, sashes, necklines, collars, skirt design and length are all factors that play into whether a dress will flatter you.

❖ Soft, feminine shapes with an emphasis on fluid lines and draping are making their presence felt everywhere, and I don't believe they are going anywhere soon. What's great is that the draped lines, soft pleats, ruching and flowing fabrics can be used to enhance and camouflage wherever necessary.

❖ The structure of these dresses is an integral part of the design, as is the choice of fabric, dress length and color or pattern. What that means is you have options galore to find a look that's perfect for you.

❖ Well designed dresses with figure flattering accents can be found by those in the know, giving you endless options to look fabulous. Wrap, sheath, empire waist, baby doll, ruched, tunic style, shirt dresses, A-line and other options make it easier to find a style that is becoming for you.

❖ Sleeves can totally change the look of a dress. Whether sleeveless, capped, short, 3/4 length or bracelet length; fitted, billowy, banded, tied, scalloped, or smocked; sleeves are an important consideration. For example, capped sleeves can extend the shoulder line, making the waist look smaller for triangle shapes or those with narrow shoulders. Sleeves with smocking, edging or other details add a softer, more romantic touch. Longer billowy sleeves add a more bohemian vibe to a dress and are great for women who don't like totally bare arms.

❖ The final factor I'd like to mention is the amazing use of color, embellishment and pattern. With more designers moving to digital printing techniques for their fabrics, a whole new world of decorative arts has been opened up and wow, it's a world of imagination, creativity, vivid colors, beading, playful design and brilliant decorative patterns. You have to be willing to get out of your comfort zone to experiment with these exciting elements. Just experiment and see whether that 70's inspired psychedelic print dress is really calling your name. How awesome if you discover it is *you*.

8) THE COAT

What is it about the longer, darker days of winter that has most coat manufacturers believe we only want to be seen in drab, somber colors like black, navy, maroon, and dark brown?

Thankfully, there are a few designers who have played with a more varied color palette and/or silhouette and designed coats that appeal to women who want to have bolder coat options.

The important points to consider when choosing a coat that suits your body shape are much the same as for a jacket, so we won't go over the same ground again.

But there are a couple of things I would like to reiterate or add:

❖ Remember, first impressions are everything. Make sure yours is fabulous, especially when it comes to the coat you're going to wear all winter. If you are
wearing a coat of any kind, it's the first item of clothing someone meeting you
is going to see. Make sure it reflects your desired style. Make a statement and
make it count.

❖ When the temperature drops, don't let your spirits drop too by wearing a drab
color that does nothing to elevate your mood. Be bold and daring and choose
a color that shows exactly who you are and how you feel; even if the weather
outside is miserable, you don't have to be.

❖ Colors that are common in the cooler months are black, navy, cobalt blue, varied tones of red and tan/beige or brown; but you can find coats in non-tradi-
tional colors like pink, light blue, olive or mustard, if you look hard enough. If
you really want to go all out, select a stylish plaid or pattern for added pizzazz.

❖ If you tend to be conservative and prefer a more understated color for your coat,
then add a colorful scarf, or a bright beret or hat in one of your power colors. As an
alternative, try a large button or brooch on your lapel to add to "eyes up" appeal.

❖ Features like epaulettes, wide lapels, a detailed buckle, fancy buttons or turned
back cuffs all add flair that set you apart from the crowd.

❖ And most importantly, buy a coat that is designed for a woman, not the boxy,
no-style , no impact variety. After all, you can still proudly display your womanly silhouette in a coat, can't you? Two words: Princess seaming!

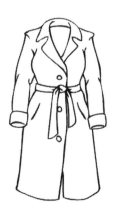

A brief note on trench coats
What man has not had a fantasy that involved a woman in a
trench (and ONLY a trench) waiting for him to open his door?
Because of our collective imagination (and those old Hollywood
movies) the trench coat exudes: allure, mystery, seduction and is
a magical mix of masculine and feminine styling.

Trench coats are the ideal 'tween seasons, coat and work perfectly
on cooler days in spring, fall, and in locales where the weather is
mild year-round.

Trench coats can be incredibly versatile and far more exciting than many winter coat styles. And they are classic and timeless. Today, they come in a range of fabrics and styles that can make them a statement piece. A red or lime green trench coat in a lustrous silk sateen says chic, sassy, sexy and savvy all at the same time, particularly if worn like a dress.

Wearing a trench gives you a glamorous look. It's hard not to feel cool and confident when you are sporting one in a great color. So go for it!

9) THE SIGNATURE HANDBAG

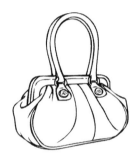

Nothing can ruin your image faster than wearing the perfect outfit you've labored over for hours with a tatty, out-of-touch handbag.

After all, isn't the choice of handbag one of the things you check out when meeting a woman for the first time? And don't you make an instant decision on the woman based on the style, quality, color and look of her handbag?

Gone are the days when your handbag had to match your shoes, which had to match your outfit. Please, ladies, set yourselves free from these tired out-of-date rules! Nowadays it's a color free-for-all; where as long as you color coordinate your handbag and shoes to go with your outfit, almost anything goes, within reason.

Your signature handbag needs to reflect your signature style; but when it comes to deciding shape, color, size, style and functionality, the key is that your handbag works to enhance your total image and reinforces the message you want to convey. After all, we *need* to carry a handbag, so why not make it an integral part of our image packaging?

The message is: choose wisely. A quality handbag is not only going to shout about the quality of your image; it's going to go the distance as well. Say no to imitation leather, overly embellished styles and cheap workmanship.

Let's now have a look at some of the important points to consider when choosing a handbag.

- ❖ Even in the most conservative environments, it's okay to play with color (if that's your thing), particularly if you favor neutral dark tones like black, grey and navy for your corporate wardrobe. A classically styled handbag in red beautifully offsets a neutral office palette.

❖ Look at your wardrobe to help you decide which handbag color will work best. If your wardrobe consists of a multitude of bright colors, then black or a neutral color is probably your best bet. If your wardrobe is predominantly neutrals, then use your handbag to add a spark of color to your look. And don't be afraid to have a few handbags on hand to give you options, some with bold color, some in neutrals. Remember handbags should be considered investment pieces. Definitely splurge.

❖ Play with shapes and decide which type of bag works best with your lifestyle. Are you a tote, satchel, hobo or shoulder bag kind of gal? Let's face it: you don't want to be switching handbags every other day, do you?

❖ Try to select a handbag that will take you from day to night with ease. Not an easy thing to achieve, but if your signature bag has class and élan, it will do it for you, no problem at all.

❖ Be sure to choose a bag that is aligned with your size and shape. For example, plus-sized women look better with square or rectangular shaped bags that don't accentuate their roundness, and that are larger in frame to suit their size (imagine a full-figured woman of average height with a teeny tiny bag—looks odd, right?). On the other hand, rectangular shaped women suit a rounded, plush bag that complements their angular frame. Petite women should really ensure their handbags don't wear them. Again it's a matter of scale. If you're small, your handbag's size should match your frame, so it doesn't overwhelm you.

❖ Choose a bag that suits your lifestyle. A busy mom probably needs a low maintenance tote that could double as a diaper bag in a crunch, is easy to clean, and offers a variety of compartments to hold all the necessities she needs to carry. A busy executive probably would lean towards a tote as well, but a sleeker, more upscale version, that reinforces her professionalism.

Like everything on your "must have" list, your signature handbag is a reflection of who you are, how you operate and the image you want to convey to the world.

Blame my mom, but I'm a big bag kinda gal. At the moment, I am using a coral/orange satchel I wear with almost everything; it contains compartments to hold all my stuff, from basics like keys, wallet, business card holder and cell phone to "Natalie necessities" like a camera, makeup, brochures, pain killers, breath mints and hand sanitizer. Now do you feel so bad about the virtual household you carry around in your handbag?

10) THE SKIRT

Don't panic! If you're a jeans and Tee gal who would rather roll over and play dead than be seen in a pretty, flowery and feminine skirt, you don't need to. We will be covering all types of skirts in a range of styles, colors and looks.

The ideal length for skirts to show off long shapely legs is just on the knee. Even if you don't believe you have long, shapely legs, this length will make them appear so.

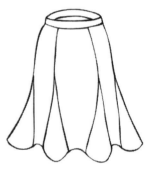

We've talked about personal style, and I explained in detail how to wear clothes that make you look taller and slimmer by enhancing your body shape. The trick is to use these tips to select skirts that are going to enhance your image and make you feel and look great.

One style that is very figure-flattering is the multiple paneled skirts often cut on the bias. They fit snugly around the waist and hips and then softly fall around your thighs and knees. This is a look that suits almost every body shape because the skirt follows the curves of a woman's body with a gentle flip at the hemline.

If flowy and flirty isn't your style, the pencil skirt is an excellent option. A straight pencil skirt that sits right on the knee is a chic, classy look.

Fabrics are a striking range of solids, tweeds, texture or prints, in either soft pastel tones or vibrant hues, which means you can choose a look that suits your style. A soft, pastel toned skirt in an up-to-the-minute print is perfect for those occasions when you feel feminine and playful. When you feel dramatic and charismatic, a textured skirt in a solid color might be perfect. Sassy? You can never go wrong with a black or red leather skirt.

Team your skirt with bronzed legs (either sheer stockings or fake tan will do the trick) to make them look extra long and luscious, and wear striking heels to add that "wow" factor.

A Word on Mini Skirts

Hello legs! Ultra short minis come in and out of fashion. But there is a fine line between looking flirty and floozy. A few words of caution.

- If you want to show off that much leg, your legs and thighs need to be in top shape. These minis are all about the legs, so if you don't believe your legs are up to it, DON'T go there!

- When there's not a lot of fabric to work with, keep it simple. Avoid detailing and too much construction.

- High heels are a must with a short skirt to keep those leg muscles taut and tight.

- Add a touch of bronzer or shimmer on your legs for a night on the town.

- Age appropriateness should be a consideration. I believe that women over 35 should tread carefully over this territory. I have seen one too many celebrities (great legs notwithstanding) who look just trashy because they are trying to rock that sky high mini way past their prime. Ladies, you just don't have to go there, so don't.

- In the same vein, there is a short threshold regardless of age. If you can't sit properly or (in the case of a mini dress), raise your hand up without showing your nether regions, your skirt (or dress) is way too short. Unless you're "working hard for your money", I suggest you don't go there either.

11) THE SUIT

If a corporate suit is part of your wardrobe, you probably have a couple in different styles and colors already. But if you don't, it's not a problem—you can easily work a gorgeous pant or skirt suit from the wardrobe basics we've already discussed.

Since we've already covered wardrobe essentials like the jacket/blazer, a pair of dress slacks and the skirt, you already have all the necessities to put together a stunning suit.

Although the concept of a serious suit may seem superfluous to your lifestyle, if you aren't required to wear one every day, you never know when you may need to attend a funeral or special event that requires the conservativeness of a suit.

How to put it all together? It's not nearly as difficult as you may think—it's all about mixing and maxing. Mix style = max impact!

The most important consideration is what impact you want to create with your image. If it's a funeral or somber occasion, it's likely you'll want an understated look. If it's a social event, you may want to upscale your look to amp up your presence.

The basic black dress slacks we discussed can be styled up or down, depending on what you team them with. A vivid jacket in a great color with complementary top and bright accessories will give your outfit "zing", while a lustrous gun metal gray constructed jacket or a black tuxedo jacket with a dash of bling will jazz up your image for evening glamour.

The same goes for skirts and jackets. If you want a flirty, ultra feminine look, team a floral patterned skirt with a jacket that picks up the tones from the print, then accessorize with matching beads or pearls. For a streamlined, professional look, team your straight or A-line skirt with a complementary jacket in any color that makes you "pop".

12) THE CARDIGAN, PASHMINA OR WRAP

When the temperature starts falling and it's that weird in-between time when the barometer can go up or down by 10 degrees without warning, nothing beats a cardigan or wrap. You can head off to work in the bright sunshine, with only a light shirt for covering, and walk outside at the end of the day to find you are freezing. So what's a girl to do?

Not to worry. These 3 wardrobe basics will help you ease into the changeable weather come spring, fall, or year round—looking fabulous and feeling comfortable.

The Cardigan
Sweater (or cardigan) sets in cashmere or light wool blend are a great trans-seasonal item because they can be layered, which is certainly a plus when temperatures fluctuate. These are classics and are here to stay and easy to dress up or down. On warm days, you can wear the tank on its own with your favorite jeans for a casual look or dress it up with classic black slacks and accessories.

Longer tunic length cardigan styles are in style lately and look great with leggings, which are very popular, or skinny jeans.

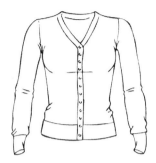

The Chanel-style cardigan is still classic, but an ultra conservative look. For more levity, there are many funky new stylings in a variety of shapes and designs. The new silhouettes are more flattering with added definition where it counts. The shorter or cropped cardigan is a new take on the classic cardigan. This looks very cute layered over a longer dress. And go wild with the variety in color choices. Try fuchsia, gecko green, fire engine red or azure blue.

A hot look is the long asymmetrical cardigan which is meant to be worn open. This is sure to stick around for a few more seasons. The wrap style cardigan is also versatile with many variations on this look available to suit your style and coverage needs.

The Wrap or Pashmina

These are a must have for transitioning into the cooler months. Wraps and pashminas are even more versatile than cardigans because you can simply slip them on or off, depending on the temperature. In addition, they can spice up your look with a dash of bright color.

Picture a simple black ensemble with a bright teal, red or purple pashmina draped around the shoulders. How fab is that? Or, if you want to bring out your animal instincts, how about a cashmere wrap in a leopard print or zebra stripe? Wow!

And the best thing about a wrap is that they're so easy to carry. Simply slip it over your arm, purse or tuck between the straps of your tote and you're all set to make a heavenly impact!

13) THE FITTED TEE, TANK OR CAMISOLE

No wardrobe can be complete without its fair share of layering pieces. And nothing, I mean nothing, is easier to layer than a fitted Tee, tank or camisole. Depending on your figure, have a selection of V neck, scoop neck, crew neck, mock turtle neck, or square neck Tees. Vary your sleeve lengths as well for maximum versatility: sleeveless, capped, short, ¾ or long. Finally, you want to have a variety of colors to choose from, so you can mix and match to your heart's content. Want to take it a step further? Get fitted Tees in prints or with details such as ruching pleating, an empire waist or texture. Now you can get really creative in your wardrobe.

You might be wondering why this item is so essential. If you haven't guessed it yet, it is one of **the fastest paths to effortless**. A fitted Tee (and when I say fitted, I mean it contours over your curves, gently hugging them) goes with everything. What to wear under your boyfriend blazer and jeans in a crunch? A fitted Tee. That cute floral print skirt you love so much in the summer looks great paired with what? A fitted Tee. You have the perfect suit but it shows a tad too much cleavage for the office. What to do? Wear a fitted Tee or camisole under it of course! You have a great wrap cardigan you want to wear but it needs, what? A fitted Tee to work. I could go on.

One of the common gaps I see when I am diagnosing a women's closet, is that she does not have enough of these underpinnings; so creating exciting new ensembles is a challenge. A wardrobe's backbone is severely weakened by a lack of items in this category. The Tee is one of the most basic "basics", which is why it is so essential.

An added bonus? These Tees do not have to cost a fortune. Make sure they are durable and have a touch of spandex so they are contouring, but this is a wardrobe must-have that you can actually skimp on. Don't buy a designer brand Tee. You're not going to get more wear out of it than the $20 version at your local H&M store or the equivalent.

A note on Tees:

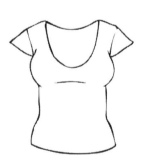

Let's be very clear. When I say "Tee", it is prefaced by the word "fitted" for a reason. I do not want you out and about sighing with relief that you can hold on to your baggy, logo'd sportswear varieties, or the ones you bought on your trip to the Caribbean and think you're all set here. No! Baggy Tees with logos are for the frumpy crowd and that's not you, now is it? If you must, hold onto sentimental pieces and wear them inside your house. But baggy Tees are not even suitable for the gym, if you're really trying to Flaunt It.

Which brings me to another important point. Some of your fitted Tees will be used casually, for exercise wear and what not. Keep these separate from the Tees you wear for your dressier occasions. You will have a pile of very casual fitted Tees for sporting, outdoorsy, exercising purposes (because we are looking cute for every occasion, right?) and a pile for your upscale casual/social occasions.

And do you solemnly promise not to slip into frumpy land by wearing a baggy, tired looking T-shirt anywhere but inside your home, or for gardening or other activities where dirt might be involved? I'm just keeping you accountable to your goal of being fabulous. Do you realize you're more than halfway there already? It's exciting!

BECOMING FABULOUS

Complete a Wardrobe Assessment

Based on the wardrobe basics we've discussed, do a thorough assessment of your closet to see which items you already have and what you need to consider adding to build up your backbone.

It's also a great time to discard any items that no longer serve you, flatter you or that are not relevant to your life, lifestyle and the new image you are in the process of creating.

Make a list of the essentials you don't already own, or those you need to update. As we continue our journey through this book, you will pick up more valuable tips and secrets about how to style your wardrobe so that you'll simply love the thought of deciding what outfit you're going to wear each day. How liberating is that?

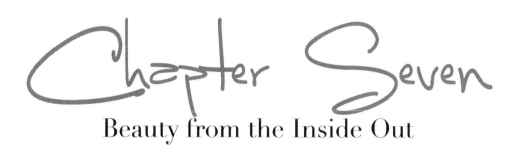

Chapter Seven

Beauty from the Inside Out

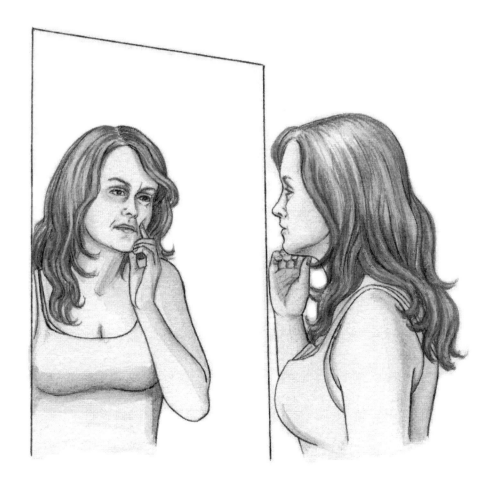

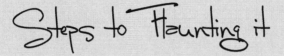

Steps to Flaunting it

✦ We radiate outwards what we feel deep inside. True beauty is about feeling confident, self-assured, happy and content. These positive attributes will then reflect outward and make you truly beautiful.

✦ As I mentioned before, you can't Flaunt what you don't feel. Feeling fabulous and Flaunting It has so much to do with our perceptions of how beautiful we are. If you consider that we are all unique works of art, how can we honestly not find beauty within us? This chapter and this book are meant to empower and inspire you to take the steps so you feel great, look great and confidently "strut your stuff".

✦ Image saboteurs are long held beliefs or ways of thinking that result in barriers or challenges to our self-images. Banish any image saboteurs from your life by first recognizing and acknowledging the power they hold over you and then get rid of them.

✦ Age is merely a number, so don't let the thought of aging consume you and turn you into an old person. Rejoice and embrace each year and learn to love the wiser, more experienced woman you become.

If you've been paying attention, you'll know for certain now how important your external image is to the way you are perceived, right? Which makes it hardly surprising that the beauty and fashion industry is so successful. Extreme makeover TV shows, the red carpet celebrity frenzy, pop culture, "What *WAS* she thinking?" articles, and unrealistic media images all focus on external appearances. It's quite frustrating to me because it gives women a distorted view of their own beauty.

Regardless of how great you look on the outside, without a positive self-image, self-possession, confidence and self-acceptance, you will not look *authentic*. And authenticity, my friend, is worth its weight in gold when it relates to how you are perceived by people. If you lack credibility, guess what? You may *look* the part, but you certainly won't be acting it.

As an image consultant, my mission is to reinforce how fabulous you feel on the inside and project this outward. It's really about giving you the tools to enlighten, challenge and educate you so you get excited by what you discover about yourself. Better yet, you will feel empowered to make the changes that will transform you internally as well as externally. And the secret of this book is that it is ALL about transformation, regardless of the starting point on your journey.

We radiate outwards what we believe about ourselves deep inside. No amount of window dressing can create true transformation if you don't like the person you see reflected back at you. The externals, as important as they are, merely enhance and refine what is going on inside. Beauty truly comes from the inside out.

THE REAL TRUTH ABOUT BEAUTY?

DOVE (subsidiary of Unilever Inc.) conducted a few groundbreaking research studies, beginning in 2004, as part of the 'DOVE Campaign for Real Beauty'[1] initiative, which highlights the impact perceptions of beauty have on self-image. Their global research project, 'The Real Truth About Beauty: A Global Report' revealed some disturbing truths, including the finding that only 2% of women around the world describe themselves as beautiful. Can you imagine? A measly 2% of the world's female population feel they look fabulous. Insanity! The study further highlighted that negative self-image is largely formed by media stereotypes.

---

1 Source: Campaign for Real Beauty Mission: www.Dove.us

Another startling study conducted by Florida Citrus Department in 2009[2], revealed that nearly seven out of ten women have avoided being photographed at special events because they felt unhappy with their appearance.

These are sobering stats.

Ladies, we have to come together to blast away these ridiculous ideals of beauty and create our own. Are you with me?

We've all heard the old saying, "Beauty is in the eye of the beholder". Some see beauty in the shape of someone's body, whether thin, muscular, voluptuous or full-figured. Others see beauty in specific facial features, while others see beauty in radiant skin, long hair, dimples, freckles, or a certain eye color. Often, it can be more intangible attributes like a great smile, an infectious laugh, a warm spirit, grace and poise or self-confidence.

What is your idea of beauty? Take a minute to think about that question and your response. And while you're thinking, consider this: based on your perceptions of what beauty is, where do YOU fit in your own beauty spectrum?

One of the things I've learned from working with women is that the way you judge beauty in others is the way you will think others judge you. In other words, if you're a person who only values facial beauty in others, you will use that same standard on yourself. Makes you think harder about your judgments, right?

Consider how your perceptions about beauty have shaped your own self-image. Imagine if you relaxed your rules about how you judged others, how much more forgiving you would be towards yourself?

This is really important, so I'd like you to ponder it long after you've read this chapter. If you're really honest with yourself, your answers may bring about a paradigm shift in the way you see yourself. And that, my dear, can be the beginning of a huge transformation. Are you ready for it?

I encourage you to think of your beauty in a whole new way, by casting a wider net around what beauty means to you. Look at yourself objectively. All of you: facial features, body shape, size, height, and all the little things that make you the unique and

---

2 Source: From the "Grapefruit Guide to Glamorous Moments Poll" Conducted by the Florida Department of Citrus. For more visit: www.GoFloridaGrapefruit.com.

beautiful person you are. If you have great teeth, then smile away. If you have great legs, Flaunt them. A strong shoulder line? A woman with beautiful shoulders can be sexy yet so powerful at the same time. Maybe you have beautiful hands? Adorn them with rings and show them to the world. You get the drift.

Whatever assets you have that you feel good about, revel in them, embrace them and make those things stand out brightly so that whatever inadequacies you feel about other aspects of your image will be moot. Focus on and enhance the positive.

We are all beautiful. Works of art, really. When you look at the entire package that is you, it is a wonder of creation. Forget about what the media pushes as the standard. They aren't real anyway. Create your own footprint and celebrate your unique beauty.

Beauty can encapsulate so many things really. It isn't just about the body you inhabit or your infectious personality. It's also about your spirit.

For me, beauty is as much about integrity, truth, kindness, contentment, as it is about my legs going on forever or the toothy smile that brightens up my entire face. I believe true beauty is timeless and age can never tarnish it.

Beauty is about being the magnificent being that you truly are! So the next time you say to yourself, "There goes a beautiful woman", or better yet, "I am beautiful", think about *all* the things that for you embody beauty: the outer and the inner aspects.

PUT YOUR REAL BEAUTY ON DISPLAY

Numerous studies have shown that it's the beautiful people who succeed in life. They get the best jobs, lead the most enriching and happy lives, don't suffer from as many illnesses; you name it and the beautiful people seem to have it!

So what's stopping you from being one of the beautiful people? We just made the case (and I hope you're on board here) that beauty isn't really just about having the perfect jaw line, a pretty nose or drop-dead gorgeous legs. Yes it includes those positive assets, but it's also about how you feel about yourself and the beauty that radiates from within.

One of the greatest joys I experience working with women is knowing I am a facilitator for change and growth. It's truly a privilege when I can help a woman move forward by uncovering the image saboteurs that may be preventing her from showing the world the beautiful woman she is.

"Image saboteurs" are long held beliefs or ways of thinking that result in barriers or challenges about our self-image. These beliefs can stem from as far back as our childhood, so overcoming them may take time and effort.

One of the most liberating and breakthrough moments you can experience on your image journey is finally conquering your saboteur(s) reaching that "aha" moment when you acknowledge it, realizing what impact it has on your self-esteem and self-image and working to blast it away once and for all.

BANISH YOUR IMAGE SABOTEURS

Let's have a look at some common image saboteurs I encounter when coaching women.

"I need to lose weight." How many of us believe we could drop a pound or two or twenty? I suggest there's scarcely a woman on earth who doesn't have that conversation going on in her head!

But for many women, the fight to attain their perceived ideal weight places them in a permanent holding pattern. "No, I won't buy those jeans until I can get into the next size down", or "I'll buy a new outfit once I've lost 20lbs". In the meantime, they let their image go. And what is the result? Nine times out of 10, their weight stays much the same, so they perpetually look like they dressed with their eyes closed!

The answer is to be happy, comfortable and confident with the person you are right now. Sure, it's easier said than done; but while you're at the weight you are, put your very best image forward.

You weigh twenty pounds more than you would ideally like to? Okay, then pump up your image and style accordingly. This book is full of tips and tricks about how to flatter your figure, no matter what shape or size you are. Use this information to style yourself so you look and feel fabulous—right now! Don't wait for that magical moment "when" or "if"… The only moment that counts is now. As the old saying goes, "Life is not a dress rehearsal", so grab a front row seat and watch the curtain rise on your show.

"My body is difficult to dress." Your body's shape and proportions are as unique as you are. Although this book describes the 6 basic body types, no two women are built quite the same. The trick is to understand your particular body shape and the proportions within it and learn the secrets about how to enhance your assets and disguise the parts you are not so comfortable with.

No one's shape is right or wrong, good or bad. Everyone is just different. Learn to make friends with your body; and like any friend, love it for its positive features and be compassionate towards those that need work. If you are a good friend to your body, it will return the favor in kind. Suddenly, you'll realize it wasn't the enemy after all—that was just in your head. Your body loves you. Love it back! And then use all the tips and tricks in this book to work the looks that best suit your body shape.

"I don't like the way I look." Many women I've worked with have a distorted or misdirected sense of what beauty means to them, or how they see themselves when they look in the mirror.

I'm no psychologist, so I can't tell you where or how these distorted reflections arise and develop. All I can do is reiterate what we previously discussed about the vast and varied dimensions that the word "beauty" encompasses and the fact that beauty is a reflection of how you feel about yourself internally as well as externally.

Why are women so much more self-critical than men? Part of the answer lies in the fact that women are judged much more by their appearance than men. And it's also because in today's society, we are constantly bombarded with images of the "ideal" face and figure. Thanks to the media, idealized images of exceptionally attractive women spread across billboards, TVs, movies and magazines have led us to believe these abnormally attractive individuals are, in fact, the standard.

The important thing to remember is that these idealized images are simply that—idealized. They are what the media would have you believe is normal, however, in reality they are abnormal—because the woman next door, or in the corner office doesn't typically look like that. This is in no way meant to judge celebrities. They inspire and motivate us to look better and to dream of glamour. Nothing is wrong with that, if it is grounded in reality. But the entertainment industry is an image based one and a distorted one at that, which does not allow for individuality or any coloring outside the lines. As women, we need to recognize this aberration for what it is and not allow ourselves to be judged by the extremely rigid and uniform standards of beauty that pervade our culture.

Only then can we learn to love ourselves for our unique and individual beauty—freckles and all.

TRANSFORMATION IN ACTION:
MEET MELISSA

Melissa is a gorgeous young woman. When she first entered my studio I thought she could be a dead ringer for Anne Hathaway. Magnificent facial features—to-die-for eyebrows, a radiant smile, the whitest teeth and dark brown doe eyes with a sparkle that was simply magnetic. She had an amazing head of luscious dark brown wavy hair. Her body, a neat hourglass. Her personality, infectious. The problem? Unbelievably, she did not perceive herself as beautiful. As a result, she dressed down, haphazardly and without intent. She had no idea what to do with her curves because, after all, if she couldn't acknowledge them, how would she know how to enhance them? She pretty much hid them in baggy clothes and unflattering sweaters.

She came to me to help her create a signature style. But as I dug deeper I realized she had a powerful image saboteur holding her back. When I mentioned that she was beautiful, she brushed it off with a remark that in her family she was the ugly duckling. I was stunned. Apparently, Melissa came from a gene pool of very beautiful women. Because Melissa did not feel that she measured up, she downplayed her looks.

When a person gets used to selling herself short, guess what happens? She begins to live in that reality, the reality that says she is not good enough. That was Melissa's saboteur. Only when she could own her fabulousness, would she move forward and Flaunt her signature look.

Melissa's "aha" moment came when she heard herself say out loud, "Well, compared to the women in my family, I am not pretty at all." Behind her infectious personality was a woman insecure about her looks. When she learned how to work her curves in clothes that were age appropriate, figure flattering, and saw the colors that made her radiate even more, a small shift started to occur. But first, she had to tackle her self-esteem issues head on.

Ladies, all it takes are those first few small shifts in perception. After that the change is exponential. When Melissa embraced her true beauty, learned how to combine her bubbly personality with her God-given external beauty, and not compare herself to anyone but herself, she started to shine even brighter.

Observation: I used the example of Melissa to show that even naturally beautiful women have self-esteem issues. The other lesson is that even naturally beautiful women can look just ordinary if they do not own their fabulousness. If you down play, make excuses, cover up—do anything to dim your lights, you will not let yourself or others see how magnificent you are. Morale: Own it and Flaunt It.

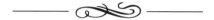

"My mother told me..." From the time we are young, we are influenced by the opinions of those closest to us, especially our mothers. And for many of us, those influences carry over into our adult life.

Did you have a dress up box when you were a child, filled with all sorts of wonderful treasures you could parade around the house in? Perhaps your box consisted of an array of dazzling hats, brightly colored dresses, gloves, old handbags and high heels that may well have belonged to your grandmother. Or like me, did you find yourself raiding your mother's closet when she wasn't around and trying on her clothes just for size? I would try on my mother's evening gowns, play with her makeup, style my hair, and look at myself in her mirror while dreaming of the time I could take the fashion world by storm.

For most of us, our first fashion icon is our mother or a mother figure, and we aspire to dress and act just like her. As we grow and change, so too do our role models and icons.

But some of us get trapped in a virtual time warp where we retain the influences and opinions that we thought were so important when we were kids. I sometimes meet women who still internalize the powerful messages about fashion and image they were taught (or not) as children. Sometimes it can be a caution as basic as, "good girls don't wear red", that may stem from our mothers' fears of us looking too sexy. Because we never understood why red is bad, we find ourselves fearfully avoiding it without even being aware of our behavior.

Sometimes the influence is much deeper. One example is the woman who said to me her mother never allowed her to wear skirts. This was a woman with to die for legs and here she was sitting in my chair and telling me she just couldn't see herself in skirts because she never wore one. Only after she started exploring why and understanding where her resistance stemmed from, could she release this saboteur's power over her.

Similarly, I've met women whose mothers' told them things about their body that impacts them to this day. Women who remark they are busty, short waisted, or otherwise unattractive, all because their mother said so, whether the observations were true or not. It's only when they see themselves in styles they've never tried and catch a glimpse of a new vision of themselves do these saboteurs start to break down. Sometimes when I am shopping with a woman she would say out loud, something to the effect of, "I can hear my mother saying my shoulders are too broad for this dress". Guess what my advice is when this occurs? Shut the voice up as many times as needed to banish the saboteur once and for all. It usually works.

To be comfortable in the skin you're in, you have to forget about the dated messages that influenced you as a child, or even as a teenager, and create your own image that is stamped with your signature style and brilliant essence. If you hear yourself saying, "I can't", ask yourself, "Why not?" If you don't have a good comeback, chances are you have a saboteur playing mind games with you. Tackle it head on.

"But I don't want to stand out." Nonsense! As human beings, we all want to be recognized and acknowledged for our unique character, personality and style.

Sure, you may not want to be the center of attention but be honest—doesn't it feel wonderful when someone notices you for your sense of poise, presence or fashion sense? It boosts your sense of self-worth and self-confidence and brings an added sparkle to you.

There's a vast difference between commanding center stage and having a signature style that makes others take note. It's not about being showy or flashy or loud or brash. It can be about a quiet confidence that radiates warmth, charm, flair and that certain *"je ne sais quoi"* that stops people in their tracks.

Some women feel that if they show too much flair, that this somehow makes them look fake or shallow. Others cherish the fact that they are naturalists, but mistakenly interpret this as a rationale to fly really below the radar with their image. Natural does not have to mean invisible or boring. And dressing with pizzazz and élan does not mean you are a simpleton.

You can stand true to your beliefs, stand out and still be fabulous you. These are not mutually exclusive things

"Who IS that woman?", they may whisper to one another. That woman is you. So allow your signature style to tell your story, bask in the radiant glow you emit and go for it.

"I am a too busy. I don't have time." I hear this comment from women from all walks of life. Whether a working mom, who invests all her time and energy into her children, or the single professional, vying hard for her next promotion, being busy shouldn't be the excuse for being frumpy. Really, the issue is not about a lack of time, but a lack of priority. Women let their image go and they know it when they do. When it becomes a priority again in their life, they take action to fix it. The next time you hear yourself saying you don't have time to shop, etc., ask yourself, "Do I value looking great?" Your answer may surprise you and may cue you in to why your image is not up to par.

"I'm afraid of unwanted attention." Sadly, for a number of women, past events, circumstances, their upbringing or life history has made them afraid to express their femininity. Instead, they hide their figures under baggy, shapeless outfits that make them look like Kansas haystacks.

It needs to be said that in some cases, the issues run a whole lot deeper than I can address as an image coach. However, for the majority of women, it's a case of helping them come to terms with the beauty of the female body in all its shapes and sizes.

Being a woman is a fabulous thing to be. For me personally, I wouldn't have it any other way. Forget whatever negative or downgrading opinions you've been fed in the past and rejoice in the fact you are all woman.

We've come a long way since the bustled, corseted, oppressed females of the early 1900s. These days women are free to be whatever and whoever they want to be and to heck with anyone who believes otherwise.

In some cases, you may need to take baby steps to gradually cast aside your misconceptions, and that's okay. Start by swapping the shapeless tent dress for a tunic top and skirt. Or take it one step further and try a soft blouse and skirt. Notice how feminine it makes you feel and give yourself permission to feel comfortable and relaxed with your new-found femininity. You'll be amazed by how looking like a woman can immediately soften and enhance your perceptions of the world around you.

Over time, you'll learn to raise the stakes and discover it feels good. In fact, it feels amazing to revel in your femininity.

"I need to be sexy to attract a mate." A number of women confuse femininity with overt sexuality and then wonder why they are sending out the wrong signals. While

it's one thing to dress to attract the opposite sex, it's a whole other ball game to dress so provocatively that becomes inappropriate. This again may stem from far deeper self-worth issues.

Whether we like it or not, we dress to impress—not just ourselves, but everyone around us, including the opposite sex. That's the nature of the human animal.

Some women just don't seem to understand there's a difference between dressing to enhance your femininity and sensuality and dressing like you charge by the hour! Many men (and most aren't even aware of this) want us to leave *something* to their imagination. Often their imaginations are a lot more risqué than anything we're likely to show them in public anyway.

We've discussed how perceptions are everything. If you don't want to be taken seriously by the opposite sex, then wearing too tight, too short clothes, and leaving quite simply nothing to the imagination is the way to get men to think you're just a play thing. And they will treat you accordingly. I know that any woman reading this book does not want that. So if you want to be treated like a lady—dress like one.

There are ways to be appropriately alluring. You can turn up the heat an extra notch by what is suggested, rather than put it on full display: a hint of cleavage in a low (but not *too* low) cut gown, a toned shoulder in an off-the-shoulder dress, the smooth curve of your tush in a figure hugging skirt or the sweeping lines of a gracefully displayed back. Smooth and subtle is going to get those male pulses racing a lot faster than overt sexuality.

When it comes to displaying your feminine charms, the rule is "understated". If you choose a low cut gown, then don't include a thigh-high split and a seductive off-the-shoulder look to boot. The key to 'understated' is to work with your signature style to create a seductive image that oozes sensuality, yet maintains mystery. Keep it classy and you'll keep the predators at bay.

"Who cares how I look?" YOU DO, that's who. And everyone you connect with cares as well. I see a regular stream of women who have fallen into such a deep image rut; they have trouble lifting themselves out of it.

These women seem to fall into two distinct groups: those who care so little about their appearance they throw on the first outfit they find in the wardrobe and that's as far as getting their image together goes. No accessorizing, no makeup, shoes and handbag that serve the purpose and that's it. Drab, drab, drab.

The other group dresses to be invisible, which can veer towards somber or fading-into-the-wallpaper. This camp is either gravitating towards dark, uninteresting hues and color combinations or neutral colors that make them blend or wash out in their surroundings. The ultimate effect is an image that is completely unmemorable with zero impact, that communicates, 'don't look at me'. Is that really what any woman wants?

Sorry gals, you may say you don't care, but somewhere deep inside you do and it's reflected in your image and presence (or lack of it). You are sending out the message: "I don't care about myself, so I don't want you to care about me either."

You owe it to yourself and those around you to look the best you can each and every day. I actively encourage you to take this philosophy on board and work with it and notice what a profound difference it can make; not only in how you look, but in how you feel about how you look.

BEAUTY AT ANY AGE

Aging is an irreversible fact of life and one that sooner or later we all have to accept, whether we like it or not. But the good news is that there are habits, tools and techniques to help us age beautifully and gracefully.

We live in an age where it is claimed 60 is the new 40, where there are such marvels in science that we have at our disposal lotions and creams to keep us looking beautiful for many decades, where wellness is the term de jour, where modern medicine can keep at bay so many ailments our grandmothers had to bear stoically, where if we exercise and eat healthy we can retain a lot of our youthful spirit and energy well past our 60's.

So what's all this ado still about women and aging?

Let's have a look at how you can maintain your inner and outer beauty no matter what your age.

_12_ Secrets TO AGING GRACEFULLY, NATURALLY

1. Age is just a number. The secret to defying your numerical age has everything to do with attitude; you are what you believe yourself to be. If you feel like an old lady it's likely you'll behave, dress and speak like one.

2. Embrace a playful and youthful attitude about life and don't sweat the small stuff. Live in the moment and for the moment. By making an attitude adjustment you can shave years from your appearance. Engage in your favorite hobbies; get active; play with children or pets; do the things you loved doing as a child; hang around with young people; spend more time outside experiencing the wonders of nature. The impact of laughter and joy in your life is powerful and it shows up in how you look.

3. Are you still dressing as if you're trapped in a time warp? If so, it's time for an image re-vamp! Grab a handful of fashion magazines and check out what the current clothing trends are. Then work those trends to reflect your own signature style.

4. Are you getting enough sleep? Most of us need between 7 and 9 hours every night. When we don't give our body enough rejuvenation time, it reflects in our face—our eyes look tired, puffy or red, which ages us instantly.

5. Sunscreen is a must. Nothing ages us faster than sun damaged skin showing up by premature wrinkles, age spots and frown lines. Take care of your skin and protect it from the sun's harmful rays. Pay special attention to your neck and hands which can be age dead giveaways.

6. Avoid cakey, thick or heavy makeup on older skin. For a makeup lift, plump up your skin with a hydrating cream foundation which softens lines and wrinkles rather than settling in them. Some of the new natural mineral powders which work as a foundation also make your skin glow: but make sure to test them at the beauty counter first.

7. Brighten your eyes with concealer under the eyes to mask puffy, dark circles. A makeup secret used by many red carpet celebrities, to brighten and open their eyes is to dab a tiny spot of ultra-light concealer or eye shadow right beside the inner corner of your eye (next to the bridge of your nose). You'll be amazed what a difference it can make.

8. No cream, lotion or potion on the market is going to get rid of wrinkles you already have, unless you opt for plastic surgery. Sorry! But you can reduce their appearance and slow the creation of new ones by using the right moisturizer. For optimal moisture, look for products that contain retinol and alpha hydroxyl acids which aid in rejuvenating the skin. There are serums that can be found in most department store cosmetic counters that deliver the most dramatic skin resurfacing benefits. Use a super-rich formula at night so it can work to rehydrate and revitalize your skin while you sleep.

9. Are you stuck in a fashion rut because you're afraid to try the latest fashion trends or you're not sure what is age appropriate? One of my clients always takes her best friend's teenage daughter on her shopping expeditions. She says that somewhere between the often outrageous outfits her teenage shopping buddy suggests and those she would choose herself, she finds a happy medium.

10. Does your hair date you? Are you still sporting the same hairstyle you had 20 years ago? A fresh, stylish haircut from a professional hairdresser can shave (excuse the pun) years off your look. Experiment with new hair colors or highlights to add luster and definition.

11. Are you wearing the right bra? A bra that lifts and supports you in all the right places can make you look taller, slimmer and younger in an instant.

12. What we resist persists. Kicking and screaming your way into another year only makes you feel worse about yourself. And guess what? The worse you feel, the worse you'll look. Hyper-focusing on every new wrinkle or grey hair only exacerbates the problem and creates more wrinkles and grey hairs. So just get over it already!

Aging is a natural part of life's journey, so accept and embrace it. Look at your crow's feet and laugh lines as sign posts to remind you of your remarkable journey and as newer, different aspects of your innate beauty.

A Final Word on our Self-Image: Every day we are bombarded by thousands of media and celebrity images that have been pinched, poked, prodded, cut, tucked, nipped, shredded, sucked, ripped or air-brushed to within an inch of their lives. So is it any wonder we mere mortals find it difficult to come up with a suitable role model who encompasses all that aging with grace and beauty embodies?

You show me a celebrity over a certain age who has allowed herself to age 'naturally' and I'll show you an increasingly rare breed of woman. Aging beauties like Lauren Hutton, Helen Mirren, Tina Turner, Iman or Diane Von Furstenberg are role models for us all.

This is not so much a judgment about plastic surgery per se. That is truly a personal choice. What I take issue with is the obsession with perfection that has invaded our culture so that normal becomes abnormal. Beauty is turned on its head and leaves in its wake, throngs of women who have poor self-images, abuse plastic surgery in the quest for said perfection, and who cannot see or own their beauty because they are so busy trying to keep up with the standard. It's truly sad. So many otherwise beautiful women cannot see their own unique perfection.

We live in a Botox culture where you really can't tell what is real. And what we risk losing along the way is the unconventional, the uncommon, the imperfection that makes us who we are—the quirkiness of a Goldie Hawn with her overly large eyes or a Barbra Streisand with her crooked nose—both beauties in their own right because of their imperfections.

I will get off my soapbox now but I think you get the point. And yes, my face is changing with age too, but often I think I am more beautiful now than in my 20's because I have wisdom, experience and self-confidence on my side. And a whole lot of sass, baby!

I have come to terms with my skis for feet (11AAA) and rail thin lower legs without a shape of curve. And you will see me Flaunting those stick legs in knee length dresses and skirts with no apology. I've been told I have a large forehead and overly wide set eyebrows. Yet the hair style I choose to rock is one that highlights these in all their glory—my hair all pulled back. My neck is longer than most and I am over 6 feet tall. My breasts are on the small side, but I honestly believe they are works of art. I have the teensiest ears, but they are kind of cute. And I have the thighs of the women in my family—full regardless of my size. All these "imperfections" make me Natalie and I embrace them all. Honestly, I would not change a thing. I didn't always feel this way, but I do now.

My wish is that every woman reading this right now can get to a point where she can say that and honestly mean it. Or, at least get to the point where she is not beating herself up because of those pesky chin hairs.

BECOMING FABULOUS

1. Look at yourself in the mirror and count at least 5 things you find beautiful about yourself, even small things like the shape of your hands or the mole on your cheek.

2. Once you've finished reading this book, take another look in the mirror and count at least 10 things you believe make you the beautiful person you are.

3. If as you read this chapter you recognized one of your image saboteurs, take steps right away to get rid of it. Whether you use a coach, therapist or the wisdom of a good book to boost your self-image, do something to allow you to put those voices from the past behind so you can move forward to being the shining star you are.

4. If you don't have a beauty routine, now is the time to think about creating one. It can be simple or elaborate, but the point is to do the things to nurture and care for your body so it ages gracefully, beautifully and naturally.

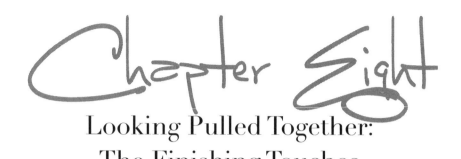

Chapter Eight

Looking Pulled Together:
The Finishing Touches

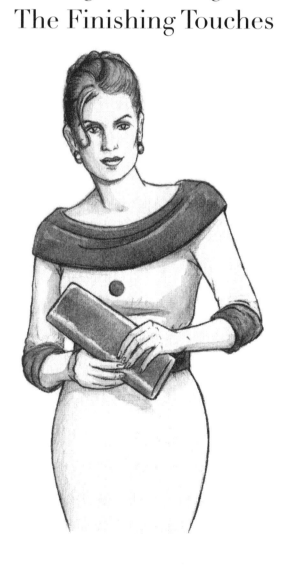

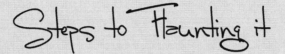

Steps to Flaunting it

- Accessories like jewelry, scarves, belts, shoes, handbags, etc. ramp up your signature look and create a pulled together, polished presence with impact.

- Use your accessories and keep building up your collection so you continue to have varied options to spice up your look. Make sure your accessories are visible when you're getting dressed so you get in the habit of accessorizing, regardless of the occasion.

- Be bold, creative and imaginative with your choice of accessories so they make a statement about who you are and how you want to be perceived.

- Makeup adds the finishing touches to your appearance, even if it's only minimal. Use makeup as a tool to make you look and feel fabulous. The same goes for your crowning glory, your hair.

- The smallest glitch in your overall 'package' creates a distraction, so make sure that ALL your accessories, from your wallet, to your gloves, to your umbrella, are worthy of you.

Wow! We've come a long way. Are you starting to feel the beginnings of transformation? Feels good, doesn't it?

By now you should have a clear vision of how to express your style effortlessly and how to dress to flatter your frame. But we still have to tackle the questions I know you have on accessorizing, don't we? After all, they are the icing on the cake.

Surely you wouldn't spend hours cooking the Thanksgiving turkey and then plonk it down on the dinner table without any of the luscious trimmings, would you? It just wouldn't be the same. And so it is with your appearance—it's the trimmings or finishing touches that can take you from looking okay to looking stellar.

PUT THE ACCENT ON ACCESSORIES

Accessories are the savvy woman's secret weapon to looking polished, glamorous, and fabulous. They are the subtle (or vibrant!) threads that pull your look together and add the finishing accents to make your creative presentation come alive. Whatever your accessory treasure trove consists of, make sure it punctuates your personal style and image.

There is an art to accessorizing that is better felt than artificially studied. Many women take a "color by numbers" approach to integrating accessories into their ensemble. These are not the women who entice you to take a second look. Rather, it is those who creatively, expressively and boldly transform their necklaces, scarves, earrings, shoes and handbags into fashion statements that work in harmony with their wardrobe. The result is a polished and perfectly executed look that makes us look twice and think "wow"! **The fastest path to fabulous: accessorize!**

For some women, it is a boldly colored cashmere scarf knotted ever so carelessly, yet effectively around the neck. For others, it's all about creating drama using statement pieces that command attention, while for some, accessories are a way to incorporate their cultural heritage into their personal style. The point is that accessories should accent, enhance, take center stage or create interest.

Here are some key accessories you can incorporate into your ensembles to help you create a pulled together look.

Jewelry

Don't be afraid to have fun with jewelry. Mix high and low, color with metal, vintage with new, costume with real.

Jewelry is an expression of your personal style and élan and has the distinctive power of blending art with fashion. It is a fashionista's insider secret, whether you are making an impression in the boardroom or the ballroom.

Here are a few more secrets to help you look fabulous with the strategic use of jewelry:

❖ Invest in a high quality watch that makes a personal statement about you. An exquisite watch immediately enhances your style.

❖ Bracelets, bangles, rings and cuffs draw attention to lovely manicured hands and slender wrists and away from upper arms, if that is a challenging area for you.

❖ Earrings help frame the face, polish your look and make a statement. They are the ultimate "eyes up" accessory. They can be as simple as pearl studs or small to medium sized gold/silver hoops or as dramatic as coral or turquoise drop or cluster statement pieces. Diamonds have great visual impact at night and are timeless. Chandelier or drop earrings instantly convey sophistication for evening wear, especially with a strapless or low cut dress.

❖ Oh, the versatility of necklaces! Like earrings, necklaces are an "eyes up" accessory which shifts the focus up towards your face. A simple strand of pearls adds a shot of elegance and panache to a classic outfit, while long ropes of pearls or chains are a very fashion forward look that also elongates your torso. Longer necklaces of semi-precious stones or beads can be worn to balance your figure because they draw attention away from hips; while choker style necklaces convey sex appeal and are great for women with long necks.

❖ Don't be afraid to mix necklaces of varying lengths, colors and/or designs together in an ensemble. If your style is Eclectic or Diva, this can be an effortless way to convey your unique creativity and command.

❖ Pins can jazz up a plain top, and when worn high on the shoulder can lengthen your silhouette. Mix and match a variety of pins for a funky, quirky look, or choose a statement piece that focuses eyes on your face and neckline. Picture a classic LBD with a cluster of colorful pins as the accent on one shoulder. Fab for sure!

Belts
Build a collection of fashionable belts. Tailored belts add polish to your look, from simple jeans and a Tee to a classically styled suit. Note the difference between a belt meant to be worn at your natural waist versus one meant to be worn with slacks—many women are confused by this. If you are aiming for a cinched waist look, you need a belt to fit your waist. They are typically made with softer leather or other material and may have an elastic back for extra comfort.

Belts are made with a variety of materials from leather and suede to metal and studs. Experiment with what works for your style sensibilities.

Remember:

- Belts wider than 1" can emphasize a trim, small waist or de-emphasize an overly long torso;

- The wider your waist, or the shorter your torso, the narrower your belt should be;

- If you're petite, be careful of contrasting colored belts which break your height;

- A dramatic belt buckle under an unbuttoned jacket can draw the eyes to the waist; and

- Don't wear a belt so tight that it causes bulges above and below the waist.

Scarves
We already touched on scarves as a wardrobe basic. They are such a wonderfully versatile accessory that can be used in a multitude of ways to accent your silhouette and your outfit. They can also be used strategically as an "eyes up" accessory.

Learn to tie your scarves in a number of ways to add pizzazz to whatever you are wearing. Long scarves slim your silhouette, while short, square scarves can be tied in any number of tailored styles at the neck.

Choose colors and prints that flatter your skin tone and coordinate with your outfit. Avoid acrylic and polyester as they will diminish your groomed and stylish image.

Shoes and Boots

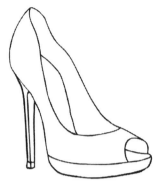

What woman doesn't have a secret love affair with shoes? The beauty of a wardrobe full of shoes is that your shoes will still look gorgeous even when you put on a pound or ten.

One of the very first things people notice (and judge you on) is your shoes, so they need to be in top shape. No scuff marks, no damaged heels, no raggedy I-just-came-in-from-the-garden styles; because by now you know the instant reaction is going to be, "This woman doesn't care how she looks".

Contrary to popular belief, you don't have to sacrifice comfort for style these days. Many designers are catching on and are more conscious about making comfort one of their priorities, so it is possible to find a fabulous pair of shoes that are comfortable as well. Designer Cole Haan has made a niche for his brand by adding Nike Air technology in the foot bed of his shoes, which gives them extra cushioning and support, without sacrificing style. Naturalizer shoes, grounded in comfort for decades, introduced a new line in 2010; its N5 Comfort series, with the goal of providing women with stylish and comfortable shoe options that focus on making the feet relaxed and properly supported. Their new technology has been dubbed "reflexology for the feet".

Another brand that is making a splash with stylish and comfortable shoes is Sofft Shoes. What I love about this brand is that even their 3" heels feel really comfortable, because again, the foot bed of the shoes are well supported. The styles are very modern, fashion forward and come in many widths and lengths for hard to fit feet like mine.

Shoe design has come a long way baby!

Want to add comfort to shoes you already own? Hit the local drug store and get yourself a couple of pairs of gels soles. Gel soles are a gift from heaven when it comes to tired arches and aching feet.

Like any accessory, shoes make a personal statement about you and the image you wish to convey. Want a polished, professional appearance? Then go for a **stylish pump** in a comfortable heel height with details and accents that suit your style. Bows, piping, stitching, buckles, embossed patterns, and animal prints are all details that can make your shoes stand out from the pack. Color plays an important role as well. For example, burgundy works well with many colors as does nude. Unless you are extremely hard on your shoes, a high quality pair of pumps will last you season after season.

Evening wear or cocktails demand a heel. Nothing brings an exquisite cocktail dress undone like a pair of flats. **Strappy stilettos** in a metallic gold, bronze, pewter or silver work well with almost any color under the rainbow, but make sure you've taken the time for a pedicure to show off your perfectly primed and painted toes.

Ballerina flats work beautifully with long flowing skirts, maxi dresses, shorts and slacks. Those with a ½" heel can even work double duty as dressier alternatives. A comfy pair of flats is also a great standby to have in the office when the high heels prove to be tough-going all day.

One of my favorite flat shoes right now is a pewter colored flat (1" heel) with a ruffle detail smack dab on the vamp of the shoe. This color can be dressed up or down and because the shoe has that interesting ruffle detail, it instantly amps up the style quotient while still being amazingly comfortable.

Sandals in the summer or warm locales are heavenly and convey effortless chic. Have on hand a couple of cute pairs whether you veer towards a thong, T-strap, gladiator style or push toes. If they are comfortable and make you feel great, that's all that counts. If you are a jeans and sneakers girl, now is the time to get fashion forward by adding these comfortable alternatives to the mix. And really have fun with the colors of your sandals. Lime green, pink, orange, purple, red, turquoise, all are good and say you are out to have fun. Don't worry about being matchy-matchy. No rules need apply.

And what wardrobe would be complete without a pair (or four?) of quality **boots**? The trend for boots in every heel height, color, style and length is not going to go away anytime soon. Want sporty? Try classic flat/riding boots in distressed leather or suede. Comfort? Look to slouchy boots that softly puddle around the ankle for a stylish alternative. Want a chic, sexy look? Then a leather knee length or higher stiletto heel boot is up to your speed.

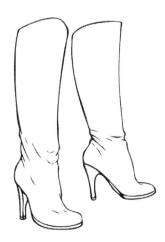

Boots can be dressed up or down and come in such a wide variety of styles that they can be worn with just about anything. Better yet, many of the quality manufacturers are widening the shaft for a roomier fit around the calf, which means no more spending hours trying to zip your boots over your ankle and calf.

Boots convey an instant fashionable vibe, especially when worn with a knee length dress or over slim fitting jeans. **The fastest path to stylish and sassy?** Boots!

GLAMOROUS GROOMING

You can undo the most fabulous ensemble if you don't pay attention to the details. Good grooming is an essential part of putting together an impeccable, effortless look.

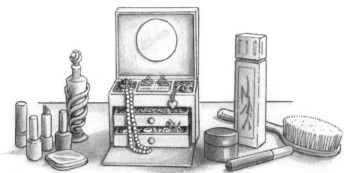

Did you know that people view us from the feet up, but remember us from the face down? So when you hear the saying, "looking you up and down", it's very real. That's why taking a couple of extra minutes to double-check ALL the details in the mirror before meeting anyone or walking out the door is critical.

Let's have a look at what I call the "3-minute scan", to ensure you are dressed to impress:

- Check that your hair is in place and don't forget to look at the back, where you will be seen more when walking or exiting a room;

- Check your teeth for lipstick stains and stray food scraps;

- Check your nose;

- Check for dandruff littering your shoulders or stray hairs clinging to the fabric;

- Check for stains on your clothing you may not have noticed when you were getting dressed;

- Check to make sure all your buttons are fastened and that all the buttons are present and accounted for;

- Check for makeup smears;

- Check your shoes for scuff marks or stains;

- If you are wearing pantyhose, check for ladders or holes;

- Check your hands to make sure they're clean, dry and moisturized (you may be shaking hands);

- If you have nail polish on, make sure it is not chipped. No nail polish is preferable to chipped nail polish;

- Check your breath. If in doubt, use a breath mint anyway; and

- Make sure your jacket is on and buttoned up before making your entrance.

To always maintain an impeccable image, keep an image survival kit close by in your car, office or tote. Your survival kit should contain all the little necessities like shoe shine, spot remover, a sewing kit, lint brush, nail file, clear nail polish, comb or brush and a mirror.

Make sure you are armed for a fashion emergency. Remember that any part of your image that diminishes your presence is a distraction from what you are saying or the work you are doing.

FACE: THE FACTS

I've spent a lot of time discussing the importance of presentation and image, and how to wear your clothes with panache, but up until now, we haven't focused in any detail on your command central: your face.

After all, your face is where all the action happens, and while I can't do anything about the features you were born with, I can certainly advise you on how to accent, enhance and enliven your face so people you meet won't be able to take their eyes off of you.

One of the questions I'm frequently asked, when I consult with women individually who don't normally wear makeup is, "But I haven't got time to apply makeup. What should I do?"

I'd like to go back one step before I answer that question. Sure, I understand and empathize with women who, for whatever reason, choose to go without makeup, however, I can't see the point in spending time and effort to give your image the impact you desire if you leave your face as bare as a baby's bottom. Your image simply wouldn't be pulled together and polished otherwise.

If I compare not accessorizing your outfit to not bothering to include the trimmings on the Thanksgiving turkey, then going without a trace of makeup is akin to not bothering to cook the turkey all the way!

So, my answer to your not having enough time for makeup, or simply not wanting to bother with makeup at all is simple: yes, you DO have time to, at the very least, add a hint of color to your cheeks, apply mascara to your lashes and a dab of lip gloss to your lips. And yes, you SHOULD bother with a subtle hint of makeup to polish and complete your look.

I never leave the house without my bare minimum: foundation, concealer, blush, mascara and lipstick. And, I've got my routine down to less than 5 minutes, so you can too with a little practice. Applying makeup isn't about looking like you're ready for the red carpet. It's about making your face like an artist's canvas, starting with the foundation (your skin) and adding as much or as little paint as you need. It starts with flawless looking skin and then adding the little finishing touches that make sense to you. The point is, it doesn't have to be this huge ordeal. Five minutes—that's all I'm asking of you. At minimum.

Thank heaven the dramatic, color-intense days of the 80s and 90s are long gone and we are now seeing a softer, more natural looking palette emerge. But perfecting the natural look that looks so…well… natural, takes a little time and effort. Looks can be deceiving: that "I'm not wearing any makeup" look that celebs like Jennifer Aniston and Reese Witherspoon embrace is simply very artfully applied makeup. A subtle bronzer to accentuate the contours, a dab of natural toned lip gloss, a hint of mascara or a gently but cleverly applied eye pencil, can lift your face and make it radiate and glow for a healthy, natural and soft effect, which has nothing in common with a drag queen. I'm just saying!

The art is in the application, so I encourage you to take the plunge and experiment if you've avoided makeup until now. Or visit your local beauty counter where an experienced consultant will show you how to apply makeup to give you the look you want.

Let's have a look at what I consider to be the makeup essentials.

Foundation

Sure, wearing foundation when you are schlepping around the house on the weekend is not essential; but it is essential if you work in a professional environment or attend an event where your photo may be taken and you need to look fabulous.

Foundation evens out your skin tone, helps overcome shiny or oily patches and sets the stage for other makeup you may apply, so you have a finished look.

Foundations come in a wide variety of formulations these days, so take the time to choose the type of foundation that best suits your skin. For even, consistent coverage, use a foundation sponge—it also saves time.

If you prefer a more natural finish (and you have the skin to get away with it), mineral powders that act as a foundation as well as a powder are great alternatives. Makeup trends go from a dewy, soft finish to matte and back again, as quickly as you can blink. My advice is to opt for the type of foundation that suits the tone of your skin and your personal choice and stick with it.

If the *idea* of foundation makes you cringe, I know you cannot protest to applying a thin layer of tinted moisturizer with SPF 30. This protects your skin and helps even out your skin tone. And yes, I've just won that little argument you're having in your head.

Blush

A dab of blush high on your cheek bones gives you a rosy glow that looks healthy and makes your face come alive. Apricot and peach tones suit warm toned skins, while pinks suit cool skins.

Start on your cheek at the half-way point below your eye and sweep the blusher up-wards following your cheek bone towards your temple. Make sure you use gentle even strokes so the blush doesn't clump, and don't overdo it. You simply want to add a gentle glow to your skin.

A trick I've taught many of my clients to use as a simple and successful makeup boost, is to brush a small amount of blush or bronzer just below their brow bone, if they don't have time to go the whole nine yards with eye shadows. It gives your eyes depth and color in one easy stroke. Try it.

Brow Business

One of the more overlooked features on a woman's face is her eyebrows. Eyebrows frame the eyes and balance your face when they are shaped and arched correctly; yet so many women seem to overlook this very critical facial attribute. They either don't shape their eyebrows at all, which means their eyes have no real 'frame' to offset them, (which gives their face an unkempt look) or they tweeze the life out of their brows, making their faces look harsh and dated. And the worst faux pas? Heavily penciled eyebrows.

Take a look at yourself in the mirror right now. Do your eyebrows flatter your face?

A lot depends on the color, shape and thickness of your brows and how they relate to your face and eyes. The perfectly framed eyebrow should begin at the same point as the innermost corner of your eye and sweep upwards to its highest point just beyond the widest part of your eye and then move downwards in a gentle arc to just beyond the edge of your eye.

Let's look at some of the key points to note when styling your brows:

❖ If you have wide set eyes, leave as much hair as practical at the beginning of your brows so that they look more close set. Also, don't make the length too long, for the same reason.

❖ Conversely, if your eyes are close set or on the small side, it's important to have as much space between the eyebrows as possible to make them appear more wide set.

❖ If you have large doe-like eyes like Penelope Cruz, don't let your eyebrows get too thick as the whole look could be too overwhelming. Conversely, if your brows are too thin, you can end up looking like you are permanently surprised, shocked or botoxed. Balance is key here.

❖ Face shape plays a role in how your brows should be shaped. Oval faces allow for a variety of shapes from a high arch with thickness or a moderate arch with moderate thickness. So experiment with what works for you if this is your face shape.

❖ Heart shaped faces require a brow with a high arch and not too much length, which can make the chin look too narrow.

❖ Long faces like mine, need a flatter brow with a lower arch to complement an elongated face. The higher the arch, the more elongating it is to the face.

❖ Brow color does not have to be an exact match to your hair; it's more important the color complements your skin tone. Your brow color can be up to two shades lighter or darker than your hair.

❖ A great way to accentuate the arch is to elongate the brow length with pencil or powder. But do so with a light touch.

Mascara

Mascara is the one tool in my makeup kit I just couldn't live without. Mascara brings your eyes to life and just opens them up so you look "bright eyed and bushy tailed". If you have fair to medium skin, use a brownish-black; if you have medium to dark skin you can wear true black mascara.

The best way to add mascara to your lashes, without it ending up on your eyes, is to look down into a mirror for your top lashes, and then apply with sweeping movements from the base of the lash upwards and out. Work from the inner corner out, and don't forget the longest lashes at the end of your eyes (for that really flirty effect).

Do the reverse for your bottom lashes—look upwards into the mirror and work from the inner corners outwards. For a big night out, or when you really want to add that "ka-pow" factor, add a second coat once the first coat is dry.

Some of the best mascaras that give you long, lustrous lashes are not the most expensive brands. If you don't want to splurge, try your basic drug store brand for fluttery, fabulous lashes.

Insider secret: Eyelash primer. This is applied to lashes before mascara and essentially primes them so they look thicker and longer after mascara is applied. If you have thin, short or sparse lashes as I do, I highly recommend primer coupled with a volumizing mascara for maximum impact

False Eyelashes: The Fastest Path to Diva!

We've all seen them: those celebs with the Bambi eyes posing demurely for the paparazzi. What's their secret? Falsies! As in fake eyelashes. When professionally done using human hair, the effect is stunning.

You don't have to be in the limelight to get the same look and it doesn't have to cost you a fortune either. Drug stores are filled with fake eyelash options, many under $10 and they're a decent quality to boot. They come in a range of sizes and styles with their own special glue for application. All you have to do is experiment with them yourself, but it does take practice to get them just right.

If you want to splurge for a gala event or simply for the heck of it, you can have lash extensions professionally applied. Costs vary from $250 upwards and they last at least a month or more. Warning, once you've seen how amazing your eyes look with a little help, you may become addicted. I recommend false eyelashes to add that "wow" factor to your makeup and to ensure your eyes are the stars every time you want to pull out all the stops.

Lipstick

Even if you demand an *"au naturel"* look, there really is no reason to go without lipstick, or at least a sheer lip gloss. Not only does a dab of lip gloss give you a finished look, it helps moisturize your lips as well.

Lipstick is a makeup staple, and over time I'm sure you've developed your own personal preferences. All the old hard and fast rules about having to match your shade of lipstick to your outfit have flown out the window. However, having said that, wearing a shade of lipstick that complements the tones in your outfit really does give you a finished appearance that has panache.

What I would like to focus on in this section on lipstick is the color red. Yes, brilliant, vibrant, luscious and oh so sexy red lipstick. One of the common denominators I encounter during my consultations is the number of women who are intimidated by the thought of wearing red lipstick, in their power shade. Nothing is sexier on your lips than the perfect shade of red.

If you are a little skittish about the vibrant reds worn by celebs like Scarlett Johansson or Christina Aguilera, I usually suggest you start out your journey with the more subtle shades like salmon or coral. What inevitably happens with most of my clients is that they get so many compliments once they "upgrade" their lipstick color, they come back to me so they can discover which shade of red is right for them. And once they've found the shade that best complements their skin tone, they look positively fabulous!

TRANSFORMATION IN ACTION: MEET CELENE

Celene is an executive who loves clothes and has an enviable collection. She knows what flatters her figure, her best colors and has a very strong sense of her preferences. But somehow she does not feel fabulous. Upon closer examination, it became clear that Celene was getting the clothing part down pat but she was entirely missing the mark on the finishing touches. She owned accessories but rarely wore them. She would leave her house in amazing outfits, but without an accessory adorning her ears, neck, or hands. She had a beautiful head of healthy hair, but her good hair days were hit or miss. Makeup wise, she had not quite found her stride, and was muddling through at best. Celene needed to apply many of the points we've touched on in this chapter to bring her beautiful outfits to life, so she could feel truly fabulous rather than frustrated, because she couldn't figure out the missing piece of the puzzle.

Celene's transformation was quick. She already had a drawer full of accessories; she just needed to wear them and not get lazy about nailing her looks with these polishing accents. She also needed to embrace a new and improved makeup regimen that made her natural beauty shine. Finally, she needed alternative hairstyles for the days when her hair misbehaved. Once we had accomplished these goals, Celene was able to start Flaunting It because she finally started to feel it.

An example of Celene's new, revamped, pulled together look would be an impeccably tailored skirt suit in cranberry, paired with a soft green camisole. Accessories would include onyx drop earrings, her crystal beaded bib necklace with hues of sage green, wine, red and emerald, her signature silver watch, a pair of wine and black croc-embossed leather pointy toed pumps, and her statement making hunter green tote. Her hair is coiffed and chic and her makeup is understated but present. The overall effect? Stylish, professional, creative, and absolutely fabulous!

Observation: Many women take these finishing touches for granted. They believe they just have to slap on a designer dress and shoes and they're done. But to be truly fabulous, women have to think of themselves as a package, where the bows and the curly ribbon are all important aspects of making the package pretty. Hire professionals if you don't know what makeup looks best on you. Get a great haircut and style that is easy to maintain, regardless of the weather, one that suits your face. And use accessories. We've talked at length about how they help pull your look together and help you express your signature style. Accessories are the fastest path to fabulous effortless style.

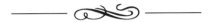

HAIR: THE CROWNING GLORY

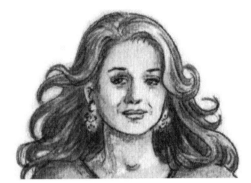

Our hair defines us as women: the cut, color, style, shine, length, all tell a story about who we are.

Have you ever noticed how a new cut, style and/or color can make you feel like a new woman? Sure, some of us are challenged when it comes to maintaining healthy, groomed hair; but if you take the time to work with a professional hair stylist, he or she can usually tame even the most difficult locks.

Although it's possible to create stunning makeup effects without paying huge prices for high-end makeup products, the same can't be said for hair products. If you have difficult to manage hair, it will pay huge dividends to invest in salon-quality hair products designed specifically for your hair type.

Your hair style needs to suit the shape of your face; so if for example, you have a round face, look for styles that lengthen your face and steer clear of straight cut bobs that end just below your ears. As a general rule of thumb, longer hair elongates your face while shorter styles, with a little contouring, can add width to your face, depending on the cut.

A good stylist can help you choose a cut that suits the shape of your face and adds personality and pizzazz to your image.

When it comes to choosing a color for your hair, make sure you select a color that enhances your skin tone. Warm, golden shades suit warm complexions while cool, ash colors suit cool complexions.

One of the biggest trends in hair styles nowadays is the use of hair extensions to add body, length and texture where you want it. The extensions can be clipped to the under side of your hair so they look natural and add instant impact. Or for that "wow" factor, you can add extensions in a different shade to give your hair the look of highlights without having to go through the whole tinting process.

Your hair needs TLC too, particularly if you use heat styling tools like blow dryers, hair straighteners or heated rollers; so treat it to the occasional hair masque or conditioning treatment for glossy, healthy hair that adds oomph to your image from top to toe.

PUTTING YOUR IMAGE PACKAGE TOGETHER

The old saying goes, "A chain is only as strong as its weakest link," and the same can be said for packaging the ensemble and image you present to the world.

I'm sure you've been here: You are chatting with a new colleague/friend/acquaintance who has lipstick smeared all over her teeth. Try as you might, you just can't stop looking at the lipstick stains, can you? Or the immaculately groomed woman you spot across the room. Her hair and face are beautifully made up. She has on a gorgeous silk suit and then… you catch sight of her shoes and they're hideous. She looks like she forgot to change out of her bedroom slippers! The positive judgments you had originally formulated are scuttled immediately because that one small point has brought her undone.

That's why I can't stress enough the importance of all over grooming, and I really mean top to bottom and everything in between. You know from your own experiences (and I'm certain you've had quite a few!) that no matter how immaculately pulled together you think you are, it can come unstuck with one miniscule detail you overlooked.

We've discussed great accessorizing to give your image added refinement and the importance of wearing makeup to enhance your appearance, but we haven't touched on smaller details that can make or break your carefully put-together image.

Consider the smaller details like a quality umbrella or a stylish wallet. You never know when it's going to rain, so don't get caught out with a less than adequate umbrella. It can be as simple as an ordinary black standard fare umbrella or a chic, feminine model, if that's what you choose; but a sudden downpour is not the time to discover your umbrella is short a few spokes, tatty or torn.

The same goes for your wallet. How many times a day do you reach for your wallet? Is it worthy of you? Wallets can quickly suffer the wear and tear of constant use, so make sure yours is conveying the right message.

Anything and everything, right down to the smallest detail, impacts how you are perceived; the quality and appearance of your hosiery, socks, gloves, cell phone case... the list goes on. Make sure that every detail is to your satisfaction.

So we've come full circle right back to where we started—your total image and what it says about you. The tiniest glitch can create a distraction to those initial impressions and prevent people from seeing you as a pulled-together, finely wrapped package in its entirety.

Make no mistake: it's the total package you'll be judged on; so sloppy nail polish, unkempt hair, a tatty wallet or a million other major and minor details will impact those judgments. What would you prefer people to think about you: "She looks frumpy and a total mess" or "She looks intelligent, fabulous and together"?

You have the power to control the image you convey and the messages you send by how well you present yourself, so you do look fabulous and not frumpy. Picture for a minute what frumpy looks like. It's not attractive is it? I don't know any woman who would consciously choose to look frumpy. Now picture what fabulous looks like to you. For every woman the image will be slightly different, but what is clear is the visual will include many of the things we've been discussing in this chapter—the finishing touches that take your image into an entirely different orbit.

And again we come back to my personal mantra, "Presence with a Purpose" ™. By practicing intent in every aspect of your appearance, you present the best possible image to the world; a powerful, purposeful and *effective* image that is magnetic. One that projects a cool, confident persona that clearly says, "This woman has effortless style. She looks fabulous, and boy is she Flaunting It!"

BECOMING FABULOUS

1. Conduct a 'wardrobe overhaul' and assess the quality of all your accessories, from your earrings and bracelets to your shoes and handbags. Cull anything that doesn't make a definitive statement about the image you want to convey. Your local women's shelter or dress-for-success organization would be very appreciative of any donations.

2. Figure out what your accessory style is. This is tough for many women and my simple advice is to experiment, experiment, experiment. Visit boutiques, flea markets, craft fairs and in–home jewelry parties for inspiration. What are you naturally drawn to? What do you dare to try, if only? I promise this will get easier with practice, but you have to put out the effort in the beginning. Look to the fashion mentors and icons you admire for more inspiration.

3. Make a list of those accessories that need to be replaced or updated and then work on gradually adding to them, so you have the variety you need to look stellar for all your occasions.

Chapter Nine

Wowing At Work

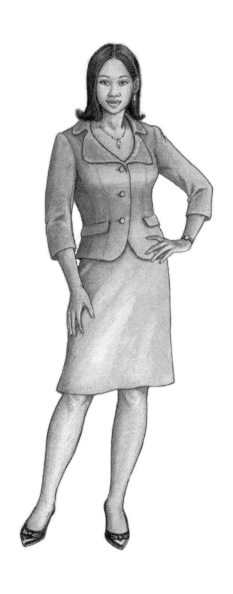

Steps to Flaunting it

➤ Women who possess professional presence exude confidence, and are seen as strategic, assertive and intelligent.

➤ Your image is an asset which can effectively position you for the success you desire. You need to successfully manage your professional image, in the same way you manage your finances or your family's schedule.

➤ Context is critical in determining what is appropriate for you to wear to work. By understanding the challenges that impact your choice of business attire, you are able to liberate yourself from being boxed in by out-dated rules or default modes of dressing.

➤ Business casual dress codes have wreaked havoc on many women's professional wardrobes. Be inspired to create interesting, yet appropriate, outfits for work that project confidence and command without being uptight or stuffy.

➤ Your work wardrobe is an investment, akin to the investment you make in your continuing education. You don't have to break the bank to build a wardrobe of clothing that is quality conscious, attractive, pulled together and stylish. But you do have to make smart clothing investments.

➤ The best way to polish your professional presence? Play to your strengths and continue to work on the areas needing improvement.

DRESSING FOR WORKPLACE SUCCESS

The whole point of the first chapter was to set the stage for all your wardrobe choices. That they be driven by intent and purpose and convey exactly who you are and what you want people to know about you. It is critical, then, that the choices you make with your business attire, are fueled by conscious intent. In this chapter, I am going to get into the nitty-gritty of dressing for work so you exude powerful professional presence.

Possessing a powerful professional image can set you apart from your peers. Imagine a woman, Ann, dressed for work with her hair in a simple ponytail, little makeup, no accessories, chinos, a dress shirt and loafers. She walks assuredly and is competent and intelligent. But she has been in the same position for over 5 years. Picture another woman, Lydia, with a chic hairdo, dressed for work in a skirt paired with a fitted jacket, sling backs, accessories and makeup. She is poised and pulled together. She commands attention when she walks into a room. Confidence, intelligence and competence are attributes immediately assigned to her because of her look. She inspires her peers and is respected by those higher up the ranks. She is a leader in her field. What's the difference between these two women? Lydia possesses professional presence, and it has helped her advance in her career.

In the professional arena, your image can enhance or hinder your goals. The question to ask yourself is this: how much effort are you willing to invest in your career wardrobe? Yes, you can be competent, brilliant, sharp as a tack, indispensible even, but if your image is not up to par with your credentials, you may find yourself being passed up for promotions, just like Ann.

This is one of those instances where it doesn't matter what is fair, but what is reality. Your image matters to those in your professional circle and the sooner you accept this, the quicker you can move on to aligning your visual presentation with your professional expertise.

An added bonus you get is self-confidence from knowing you look exactly as you intend. But even better, is the changed perceptions about your professional abilities from those around you. This can suddenly open doors for you. I'm not talking abstractly here. I've seen this scenario repeatedly with women I've worked with.

Why aren't more women dressing to impress at work then? Many of today's professional women lack the time and wherewithal to create the polished and pulled together office outfits they desire, to meet the demands of their careers. This is why so many women resort to uninspired "defaults", including: the traditional suit; black slacks and a sweater; chinos and a button down; jeans and a button down; or some variation on these. In their minds, it is better to blend in and play it safe rather than risk making a gross wardrobe faux pas.

What's missing in these women's work wardrobes is a happy medium. Heck, what is missing is a big dose of personality. These may be women just like you. This might very well be your story too.

If this is you, regrettably, style and presence has gone out the door and with it, your opportunity to shine, not just in the caliber of your work, but in your visual presentation. Remember, your image is your packaging of YOUR unique brand. If you're dressing in "default" mode, your attire is not going to represent you at your most brilliant. It certainly won't help you look or feel empowered, confident, polished, fresh, modern or *present*. It will most definitely not have "intent" at its core.

I know it's not that you don't care about how you look. It's that you are simply uninspired to do better.

STRATEGIES FOR A WINNING WORK WARDROBE

Context is so important in determining what is appropriate for you to wear to work. Are you in a corporate or informal environment? Do you own your own business? Do you telecommute? Does your company have a dress code policy? What are the women senior to you wearing? What type of industry are you in? What is your role? Are you in the public eye? What outfits makes you feel most confident? Where do you work? Snazzy boots and skinny jeans may work in a creative office environment in New York City, but can be career suicide on the Hill in Washington DC. The key is to be smart about your career wardrobe, no matter where you work or what you do.

Remember: *people are going to make at least 12 assumptions about you based entirely on their perceptions from the image you project. And they are going to make those assumptions in less than 30 seconds.* Your goal is to perfect the art of presenting a powerful, polished, professional presence--the FIRST TIME, EVERY TIME. This way you can be ensured your image is working for you.

Many of the principles we previously discussed to help you look fabulous in other aspects of your life also apply to looking fabulous at work. However, most women don't approach their work wardrobe setting out to look fabulous—they just want to be professional and appropriate. Don't worry, I get it. But we can achieve all these goals and more, by shifting our perceptions of what is professionally appropriate, given our work environment, role, industry, and context.

I realize this can be confusing given the many variables in play here. Let me spend some time breaking down some of the scenarios you may face as you decide what your work style needs to look like. We're going to use these scenarios as a way to illustrate the main points that reflect the challenges you may encounter as you dress for work. Perhaps you can relate to one or more of the following eight scenarios of **Wardrobe-Challenged Professional Women**.

1. **ANDROGYNOUS:** You work in a very casual environment and most of your peers are men. You want to fit in, so you likely suppress your femininity and dress like one of the guys. This could look like a polo shirt, chinos and flat shoes. You are bored by your work attire and know it doesn't become you. Yet you have no idea how to blend in while still expressing your softer side.

2. **SUIT SETTLER:** You work in a corporate environment which used to be very conservative. You were comfortable in your suit, pantyhose and pumps. In recent years, the dress code has become more relaxed and the women around you have updated looks and styles that surprise you. You struggle because you feel the new dress codes are too relaxed for your tastes, yet you know your suits make you appear uptight and out of date.

3. **MUSE INTERRUPTED:** You work in a creative field where expressiveness is encouraged. Yet as good as you are expressing your creativity at work, it does not translate to your wardrobe. You impulsively buy unique accessories and clothing, yet you don't know how to pull them together in a cohesive way. You angst over what to wear each day as your work style is not clearly defined. You resort to play-it-safe separates that leave you feeling out of place and out of sorts.

4. **POWER PLAYER:** You are a leader in your field. Perhaps you might own your own business. Regardless, your clothing needs to reflect the power player that you are. But other than the traditional dark suit and a button down, you're not sure how else to project your authority. You are afraid you will not be

taken seriously as an executive if you dress in a way that is more expressive. Your work clothes are safe, but at least you don't risk your work status for the sake of style.

5. **WALL FLOWER:** You want so much to blend in. Your work wardrobe consists of various basic black pieces you mix and match. You want to get out of this all black and boring rut, but are scared to truly stand out for fear you will wear the wrong thing. So you continue to be invisible, risking career advancement in the process.

6. **ONE WOMAN SHOW:** You may own your own business or be in the public eye. You wear many hats in your business: some days you may be out and about meeting with clients/customers, other days you may be attending a business luncheon or chairing a meeting, and once a week or so you're running around doing errands for your business. You need your work wear to serve myriad occasions and contexts. But you have no time to keep up with the demands of your work attire. Figuring out what to wear each day is a challenge that you meet with a hodge-podge of favorite pieces that you wear over and over. You struggle with being on the go, yet still presenting a polished and pulled together image.

7. **BORED WITH BLAH:** You telecommute, but every two months or so you have to attend a meeting at the office. You dread those days because you have no idea what to wear. You're not in the office regularly enough to observe what your peers wear and your own personal style is very relaxed. You end up wearing your "uniform": slacks and a button down, with the same black jacket. You know you can do better, but have no idea how.

8. **PRACTICALIST:** You need a functional, practical wardrobe because of the nature of work you do. You find yourself dressing in comfy jeans and easy tops. However, while practical, they do not scream "career woman" which leaves you dissatisfied. You need to elevate your work look, while wearing functional clothes that are inexpensive that you can run around in. You have ideas of outfits in your head, but they don't translate well upon execution.

While these are just a few examples, I'm sure you can relate to at least one of these scenarios. If dressing for work is challenging for you, I want you to understand that you are in good company. Other women share the same fears and challenges about workplace attire.

Since you spend so much of your adult life at work, shouldn't you at least be satisfied, if not thrilled, with your attire while working? I believe you absolutely should. It will impact the way you feel, the way you walk, your level of confidence, and so much more.

To help you address the dilemmas above, I'm going to revisit some principles we covered in earlier chapters. However, the focus now is on applying these to your business attire, so the advice is much more targeted to your work life. I'm also going to cover new ground here, so stay with me.

You can begin to incorporate the guidelines below into your work look to present a sharper, more cohesive and impactful image. Let's give it a whirl, shall we?

Accessorize

In Chapter 8, we discussed accessorizing as one of the simplest ways to elevate and pull together your look. This is especially the case for your business wardrobe, as your clothing options may be more limited than your non-business wardrobe. The right accessories can pretty much address all the scenarios above. For women needing comfort and practicality in their wardrobes, adding a colorful scarf tied in an unusual way, a belt at the waist or hip, a statement handbag and stud earrings can immediately make your 'basic' outfit look infinitely more interesting. For women who need more flair in their work wardrobe's, upping the ante with statement making jewelry, killer heels, textured, patterned or embellished scarves and a handbag or tote that commands attention, will help your style go the distance, regardless of where you work or what you do.

For work, remember to stick with one main accessory. If you're rocking a bold necklace, your earrings should be very demure. If you're flaunting a funky leather belt, then you want to tone down the necklace or opt to not wear one at all. It's ultimately about balance.

The beauty of developing an enviable collection of accessories of different lengths, styles and sensibilities, is that they are a great way to spruce up your work wardrobe without breaking the bank. They're also a fabulous way to express your personal style, while still being work appropriate. Use your new knowledge of your burgeoning personal style to find accessories that help you reflect your sensibilities at work. You can wear a classic suit and pair it with a show stopping neckpiece and command even more attention. That simple shift can be transformed into an interesting and dramatic ensemble by coupling it with the right necklace and skinny belt. And if your work wear is on the relaxed side of the spectrum and needs a boost, adding accessories takes your look up several notches instantly.

The work accessory that never let's you down regardless of where you work or your style sensibilities? A stellar watch; practical and functional but absolutely the hallmark of professional sophistication. Refer to Chapter 8 for more ways to accessorize your work wear with confidence.

Necklaces

I know a necklace is an accessory and we just discussed those. But these beauties can have so much impact on your work look, that I think they warrant their own category. Necklaces are instant "eyes uppers" (yes, I've created a new verb). An easy rule of thumb is to select necklaces that mirror the necklines of your outfits. But there is added interest in contrasts: if your neckline is high (crew or bateau, for example), a longer necklace will create a focal point lower down on your torso. This is a great way to accessorize a simple sheath dress. If you are showcasing more of your décolletage, a necklace that sits front and center near your collarbone is a stunning accent. Consider the color of the necklace and how it works with your look. Adding a necklace in a contrasting color can jazz up an otherwise boring suit. If you're aiming for a more signature vibe, combine necklaces of varying lengths, stones and metals in one outfit can truly make a look your own.

A bib necklace that sits neatly on your collarbone adds instant oomph to any outfit. This is an effective tactic when your neckline is plain and you want to add more drama or edge to your look. The bib necklace is statement-making by default and when it coordinates well with your outfit, blends in seamlessly so you look like you have created a completely new neckline. Make a Romantic statement with a flower embossed bib design or a Diva one with an edgy abstract or architectural design.

A growing trend is to add brooches to tiered necklaces in a mix and match way. This really works for women who are very expressive or want to project an Eclectic sensibility. It is the ultimate 'build-your-own-necklace' project and makes a unique, fun and creative statement to your otherwise basic business attire.

Color

For those of you with very drab work wardrobes, slowly starting to incorporate color into your outfits can instantly aid you in stepping that much closer into the spotlight. Color can be added in myriad ways: a burst of cranberry from a fitted T-shirt or tank, a splash of sienna from your scarf, a glint of sky blue from the stones in your necklace, or a dose of forest green from your jacket or cardigan. It all works ladies!

Remember what you learned in Chapter 2 about using color strategically? A few quick reminders: Dark colors such as black and navy blue convey seriousness and authority; brown, while professional, has less authority than black or navy but it engenders reliability and security; pastel colors are soft and convey approachability and femininity; red communicates strength, confidence, command, assertiveness and a touch of daring; every neutral can be paired with another neutral; grounding bright colors with white makes them pop; and pairing black with bright colors tones them down. Feel free to wear your best colors year round.

Print/Pattern/Texture

For women who are willing (or need) to push the boundaries of their business attire further, in addition to color, you can add interest and élan to your work look by mixing in print, texture and pattern. These elements can be mixed into your ensembles *quietly*, as in the leopard print skinny belt you cinch your waist with, the pinstripes in your fitted shirt, or the croc embossed texture of your shoe or handbag. They can also be added more *loudly*, as in the floral pink and grey pattern in the blouse under your jacket, the hounds tooth brown and ivory jacket you pair with your slacks, the paisley swirls of your favorite wool scarf, or the eclectic geometric print of a skirt.

The point is, you will ultimately determine how much to turn up the volume when integrating these elements into a particular look. But the volume needs to be audible. You hear me?

A question I am often asked is how to work with different patterns in the same ensemble. This definitely is an area that takes experimenting and is best suited for women who are more confident about their fashion choices. But generally the trick is to consider scale, line, shape and color when you are mixing pattern with pattern. There should be some common element(s) that draws the patterns together. Imagine a navy and white polka dot dress pulled together with a blue and white striped belt. Two different patterns but the colors marry the two. Similarly, picture a grey and pink circular geometric patterned skirt paired with a black jacket and accented with a pink, blue and white floral scarf. Imagining this outfit as a whole, the jacket grounds the look and the rose print on the scarf and circles on the skirt mesh with each other. Can you visualize it? Don't get me wrong, mixing patterns in this way is not for everyone or every work environment. But if you want to make a show stopping statement with your look, this is a creative way to do it.

Structured/Fitted Jacket

The structured or fitted jacket can address a multitude of workplace dilemmas. It is the ultimate work wardrobe staple that belongs in every career woman's closet. The sharp contours of a jacket immediately projects command, authority and power. But make no mistake, we are not talking about a boxy, wimpy or traditional suit jacket variant here. One word ladies: Silhouetted. Whether you couple your jacket with a blouse, shirt, turtleneck, knit T-shirt, or camisole, it has to fit your body like you are a woman. I know that "menswear inspired" is a trend that repeats almost ever year, but please don't take that term too literally. That is, unless you're *really* going for a more manly look, which is a different matter entirely. Try to train your eye to look for the details that make a jacket contour to your body.

What details? You know, the ones I keep repeating throughout this book: cinched or belted waists; princess seaming in the front and back so the jacket skirts over your curves; peplum styles that create an hourglass look even if you have a rectangle figure; lapels that lay nicely on your shoulders; designs that create contours such as peaked edges; low stance buttoning that creates a deep V in the center of your torso which minimizes your waist; and, subtle shoulder padding. Those little details make the difference between you looking like a stand out AND in charge, versus being just another 'suit', or worse, invisible.

Structured Dresses

I would be remiss to go on and on about the structured jacket without giving a generous nod to the structured dress. First Lady Michelle Obama was not labeled the "Commander in Sheath" by Vanity Fair when her husband was on the campaign trail, for nothing. The sheath dress is the quintessential classic structured dress that Jackie O made one of her signatures, decades before Michelle Obama made them her own as well. Sheath dresses are a softer, more feminine and more accessible variation on a power suit. A sheath dress can be paired with a jacket or longer topper to create a knockout professional ensemble that still reeks of power and confidence.

This is a perfect solution for women who need to mix things up so their work wardrobe expresses more pizzazz, while still erring towards the more professional and conservative end of the spectrum. Sheath and other structured dresses come in a variety of colors, prints and silhouettes. The critical elements are that the dress is fitted without being tight, generally has a modest neckline, and falls at the knee or an inch or so above or below. Many of these dresses are designed with inset waistbands so the waist is showcased. Asymmetric necklines are popular with some designers and this adds a slightly fashion-forward vibe to an otherwise conservative dress. The dress can be sleeveless, capped sleeved or ¾ length sleeved. Women in more relaxed work environments should look for designs with interesting accents or details and can choose to pair the dress with a cropped cardigan or wear solo. Styling with accessories, including brooches, earrings and necklaces can bring even more joie de vivre to this look.

If a sheath dress is not figure flattering on you, don't despair. A trench style dress with an A-line skirt is a great structured dress option. The collar, sleeves, buttons and pockets all create *structure* to the look so there is no mistaking who is in charge. Keep the color in the darker hues for optimal command.

Quality

Your clothing can be one of your most important career 'investments'. Look for timeless, well tailored designs and mix these up with stylish accents that suit your personality. Wear only what fits you perfectly. Have your clothing altered by professionals as needed, and pay attention to the designers and brands that work well for your proportions and figure. If your $1,500 Max Mara suit puckers in all the wrong places, you're better off wearing a cheaper alternative that fits you immaculately. Remember: nobody sees the labels.

The fabrication of your work wear is important if you want your pieces to exude success and if you want them to work for you for many years. This is important for *every* professional woman. Cheap fabrics lessen your credibility, no matter how cute your outfit might be. Again, you don't have to spend a fortune to find well made, quality work wear. But you do have to learn how to spot them.

Here are a few important details you should understand:

- **Lining**. Whether you have your mind set on purchasing a jacket, pair of slacks, dress, skirt, or suit, a garment that is lined will always drape more flatteringly over your figure than an unlined one. Lined pieces fit you better, last longer, and are a clear sign of quality workmanship.

- **Fabrication**. Natural fibers such as wool, silk, leather, linen and cotton are generally great investments, but don't be fooled into thinking that they are all created equally. As expensive and luxurious as cashmere is, it is infamous for its questionable durability. Pure cashmere will eventually 'pill' (get those little fuzz balls on it) and when that happens, in the discard pile it must go. Cashmere blends are more forgiving. Pure linen is lovely but it attracts wrinkles. Most quality linen suits are blended with another fiber, such as cotton or silk so they can stand up to a day's wear.

On the other end of the spectrum are manmade fabrics such as polyester, rayon, and microfiber. Before your mind starts thinking of the 70's polyester suit, hold on. Polyester, microfiber and rayon blends can be fine if they have a substantive drape, are blended with other fibers and are well made. You can find suiting made of a Polyester/ Rayon/Lycra blend, possibly at every price point.

The truth is there are no hard and fast rules about fabrics anymore. I find that observing how a fabric drapes on your body, and looking at the detail of its construction, are some of the best measures of determining whether it is worthy of your investment.

- **Hardware**. A surefire giveaway that your jacket is inexpensive is the quality of its buttons. Cheap buttons, zippers, grommets, or snaps diminish the quality of your garment. If you love an item but hate its buttons, you can easily replace them to instantly upscale the piece with the help of your new best friend, your tailor. Note: Most quality garments come with their own spare buttons sewn on the inside seams.

- **Drape**. Flimsy pieces do not scream "I'm a woman in charge!" Any garment that is see-through, hangs poorly on your body, stretches after the first wash, or looks like the strongest wind gust will whisk it away from your body (hello wardrobe malfunction), is probably not suited for work.

Consider the quality of all your business accessories as well. This includes not only the accessories we discussed above, but in addition, your laptop bag, wallet, business card holder, portfolio case, umbrella, lipstick holder, et al. At any time, any one of these items can come under scrutiny and that polished image you have been cultivating can be whacked away in one fell swoosh of a tattered handbag.

SLACKS, SKIRTS AND OTHER WORK WEAR BASICS

In Chapter 6, we covered great depth discussing your wardrobe's backbone. Now I want to zero in on a few critical pieces that will help relieve some of the stress you have when deciding what to wear to work. Whether you are having a casual business lunch, clocking it away at your 9 to 5, meeting with customers or clients or doing any of the myriad tasks your career demands of you, these pieces are "backbones" for every career woman.

- **Trousers.** At the office, a classically cut trouser is much more professional than a fitted pair. When in doubt, opt for a straight or full leg. If you're tall, you can even choose a palazzo pant (more flare in the leg). Charcoal grey is a wonderful color in lieu of black and it is softer with other colors it is paired with. Imagine a saffron hued wrap jacket paired with dark grey full leg slacks. This is an unexpected color pairing, but absolutely work appropriate and every much a power play as a matched suit, without the added formality.

- **Cardigans.** Cardigans are an effortless way to revamp your work look while still rocking a relaxed vibe. The variety of styles that abound also makes it easy to find your fastest path to figure flattery. The cropped cardigan is a wonderful way to add a layer over a dress or top without overpowering. It's also a cool way to add a jolt of color to a neutral ensemble. The tunic length cardigan is a great relaxed look that you can belt, wear open like a topper or button through the middle over slacks or jeans. The asymmetrical patterned cardigans are fun and add levity to your work wear without compromising your professionalism. More classic tastes can enjoy the traditional hip length cardigan paired with a skirt for timeless appeal.

- **Skirts.** Speaking of skirts, the pencil skirt has become iconic at work. Its clean lines and classic sophistication are definitely winners. There is something about its contained vibe that signals both pulled together and all business. Yet it is also sexy because it showcases curves. Whether you opt for the retro styles with higher waistlines or those that fall closer to your hips, this skirt is most polished when you tuck in your blouse, shirt or sweater. Alternatively, you can pair with a peplum jacket or slightly blousy top that falls just below your belly; the trick is to keep the skirt's sleek silhouette intact. This is a great option for curvier ladies or those with a tummy poof.

But let's not give the A-line fit and flare skirt, short shrift. This is a work wardrobe must have, particularly for those women who are bottom heavy or plus-sized. To anchor this style of skirt, pairing it with a more structured jacket or shirt will project the professionalism desired. For work, skirts at the knee or just below are most flattering. Back in vogue are the midi length skirts that fall just above the calf. These are a fine alternative for work if you make sure you pay attention to your proportions. Generally, you will want you jacket or top falling around your hip or higher with this length skirt for optimal figure flattery. Maxi skirts are tricky at work because they tend to convey a more bohemian sensibility. If you work in a creative or very relaxed environment, they are worth a try if you tame their ethereal vibe with a fitted jacket, or knit top.

- **Dark wash jeans.** For those in casual work environments, jeans can be appropriate. They should be trouser cut, which has a fuller leg, so you keep your lines clean and your look appropriate for the office. Minimal to no detailing or embellishment is best. A higher rise is also more comfortable for most women and also more appropriate for the office (no un-intended peek-a-boo's), so look for waistbands that fit around your navel. You'll want at least 2% Lycra in your jeans for fit and comfort. The "give" in the stretch ensures that the jeans won't sag or pucker by day's end. Dark blue, grey, black or dark brown are great choices. I don't recommend skinny jeans as a work staple, except perhaps for the woman on the go, or those who work in creative fields, where there is a need to be trendy and fashion-forward for work.

- **Knit tops.** Your work wardrobe would not be complete without a staple of knit tops to fill in the blanks when you need an easy go-to look. Stock up on these in your best colors and try adding some print and pattern too for extra pizzazz. Knit tops can be worn practically year-round and have more presence than a fitted T-shirt, because the fabric is more substantive. Wear solo or mate with a jacket or cardigan depending on the business occasion.

- **Shirts and Blouses.** All women can add a few of these toppers to their wardrobe to project easy, effortless style that is still low maintenance. Look for interesting accents such as bow ties, ruffles, pintucking, ruching, seaming, zippers, sashes, and unusual necklines to make these tops stand on their own merit. Again, work with your optimal power colors for the most impact. Consider wearing a camisole or tank inside your top or cinching with a belt for alternative looks. Of course you'll want to layer with a jacket or cardigan as the occasion warrants, as well.

- **Vests.** These are a fun way to add structure to a blouse, shirt or knit top. Vests lend a certain formality to your look, but are more versatile than jackets, making them a great choice for less formal office settings. Vest should be fitted so they contour with your figure. Keep the colors on the neutral end of the color spectrum so you can blend your vest easily with other pieces. Layer over sleeved tops of different colors and styles for many creative options. Take a cue from menswear, and couple your jacket with a vest instead of a traditional top for an authoritative look that has a dose of sass. (Note how I rock a vest on the back of this book!)

- **Shoes/Handbag.** Refer to Chapter 6 for guidance on how to make sure your footwear and arm candy are worthy of your career aspirations.

I hope you're breathing a sigh of relief right now. It's not as hard as you thought, is it? You can rock it out at the office and take no prisoners while you're doing it, regardless of the scenario that most challenges you. Maybe after reading this section, you've discovered that you can still wear your power suits but you just have to add flair with accessories and accents. Perhaps you've realized you can elevate your relaxed look without sacrificing comfort, and without blending into the woodwork. Maybe you have been inspired to be more expressive with your work wear choices, so your image really reflects the type of work you do or the field you are in. It's all good.

While this information is by no means meant to be an exhaustive career style guide –the types of work, clothing choices and scenarios women are faced with these days are so diverse—it is meant to inspire you and motivate you to make needed changes.

I have an atypical work wardrobe, as I am a business owner in a creative/ fashion field who is almost never in an office setting. My work wardrobe scenario is closest to that of the "One Woman Show's". If I am shopping or doing a wardrobe audit with a client, my wardrobe tends to be more relaxed so I can move around easily. I am still accessorized, pulled together and modern in my look, but I am practical. If I am conducting a seminar on "Presence with a Purpose",™ then of course I am going to wear a jacket and a coordinating skirt or slacks, or a professional dress. Matched suits have never been a preference of mine and I am not mandated by anyone to wear one, so I don't. When I am networking, I can get very professionally expressive with my attire because I want to look distinctive, to stand apart, and to make people say, as they often do, "You are a great brand for your business." I choose to express my sensibilities the same way I encourage you to express yours. Context, like I mentioned in the beginning of this section, is fundamental.

CAREER INSPIRED ENSEMBLES

To help give you even more inspiration, below are **8 different work looks** (that do not include a traditional matched suit—you already know how to do that!) that suit different work environments, and contexts. These illustrations veer more fashion-forward and are meant to push the envelope a tad. After all, to inspire you, I have to get you outside your comfort zone. Use the illustrations as muse, and as a way to start defining new ensembles that could work for you in the professional arena, that also convey your unique style sensibilities.

As you consider the possibilities, remember that your work wear includes the occasions when you are networking, attending a business lunch, participating in happy hour with your colleagues, meeting with your clients, and more. And trust me; I'm not knocking the traditional suit. This chapter began with an illustration of a woman rocking a traditional skirt suit. Suits have their place and context and are easy to put together. I have utmost confidence that with your knowledge of figure flattery and personal style you can find suits that make you shine. It's the other hybrid ensembles where most women need to flex.

Use these looks as encouragement to take your business attire into another orbit!

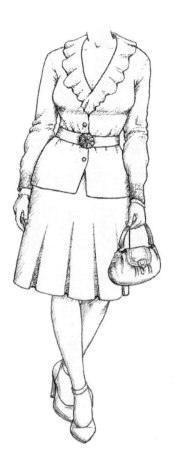

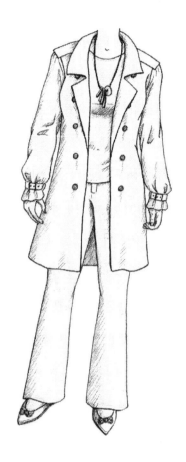

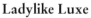

Ladylike Luxe

This is a great choice for women with more Romantic sensibilities. This is also a very forgiving silhouette for many figure types. Because it is perfectly business-appropriate it is a stellar ensemble for Suit Settlers, Power Players, Bored with Blahs, and One Woman Show's.

Casual Cool

This lightweight trench worn as a topper over slacks is as simple as it gets, but it still packs a powerful punch. Modern, effortless and still commanding, this should be a go-to for Androgynous', Practicalists, Bored with Blahs and Wallflowers. Muse Interrupteds just need to add jazzier accessories.

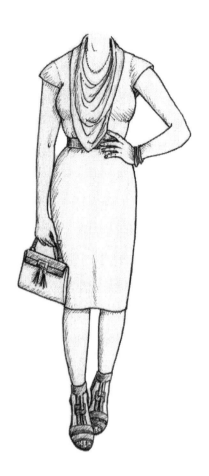

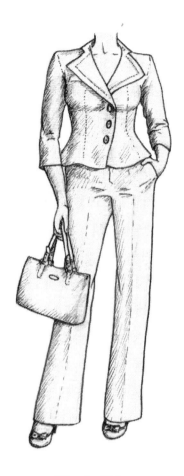

Polished Panache

Classic Chic

This cowl neck, belted dress screams Sophisticate with just a touch of edgy. This commanding yet feminine look is perfect for One Woman Shows, Muse Interrupteds, and Power Players. Tone the shoes down a tad and it is a fresh alternative for Suit Settlers.

You can still flaunt the look of a suit with separates that stand on their own, like this peplum jacket and slacks. This is an all business look, but oh so modern yet classic too. This ensemble is a great option for Suit Settlers, Power Players, One Woman Shows and Wallflowers.

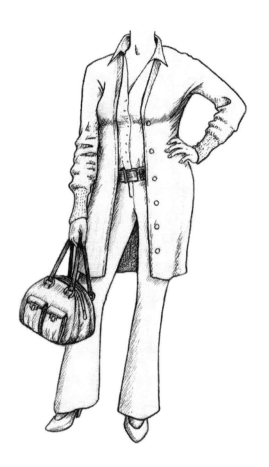

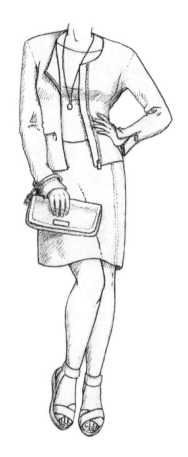

Comfy Confidence

Subtle Sassy

A comfortable outfit does not have to be boring. This tunic cardigan and slacks outfit conveys an easy pulled together look. This is a wonderful choice for Practicalists, Bored with Blahs, Wallflowers, Androgynous' and One Woman Shows.

Easy-breezy and feminine is the vibe of this jacket and straight skirt. This makes it the perfect solution for Wallflowers, Androgynous' and Practicalists. Swap out the sandals for boots or pumps for a more conservative look for Power Players and Suit Settlers.

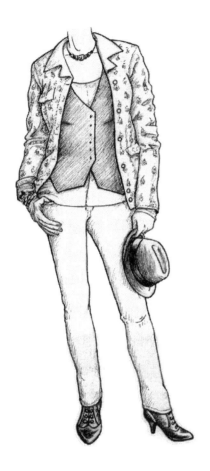

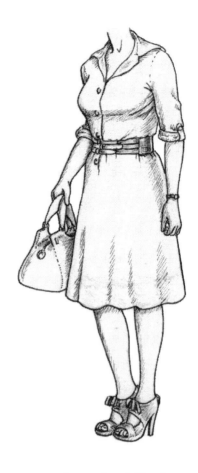

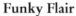

Funky Flair

This very expressive look has a strong Eclectic underpinning. It is perhaps the most aspirational look for Muse Interrupteds. This look could also work for One Woman Shows and Bored with Blahs depending on the business context and industry.

Everyday Effortless

The classic shirt dress never fails. What keeps this from looking boring are the attention-getting accessories it is paired with. This look is a no-brainer for Practicalists, Wallflowers and Androgynous.

RELAXED DRESSING AT WORK

A question I often get from women regarding their business attire is how to convey a commanding and authoritative presence while not losing touch with their femininity. This is a great question. The age where women HAD to wear power suits to exude success is pretty much over. Often women seek my expertise because their version of a power suit has become their "uniform" and they want updated options that are more relaxed, but equally as impactful.

In many professional environments, business casual dress codes are the norm. Relaxed dress codes were originally designed to help employees....well, relax! No more restrictive power suit, panty hose and pumps (sorry "Suit Settlers"). Thumbs up, right? Well, not exactly. Business casual wear has actually caused more anxiety and confusion for many women who now have no clue what to wear to work.

Women focused on their career often don't spend time perusing fashion magazines. They're used to putting a suit together—just add a blouse and voila, work attire. Throw business casual into the mix and you get what I like to call, clothing "noise" –way too many options. For the career woman, whose time is already fragmented, figuring out how to put different "professionally appropriate" ensembles together often is a new and unwelcome challenge.

I see women struggle with this too often. The great news is that once women understand the boundaries of casual versus professional wear and are informed about the options that suit them, they can begin to approach dressing for work more effortlessly.

I'm here to offer you help if you work in a business casual environment and are stuck in a rut. Below are a few guidelines to help you navigate this fuzzy territory.

7 Winning Ways TO WOW WITH BUSINESS CASUAL

1. A business casual ensemble is one that is still polished, yet not so uptight or rigid that you look like you're ready to chair a meeting.

2. A good rule of thumb is that business casual wear typically means mixing an informal piece or two into classic pieces so you can express your style with élan. So it's "relaxed" yet still pulled together.

3. Summer is a notorious time for women to get too relaxed with their dress and this is especially true about the shoes they wear. Flip flops run rampant. Any shoe that can pass for a slipper is a "don't" in a professional context. The same goes for any shoe that looks like a variant on a running shoe. What is appropriate? Your standard pump, slingback, peeptoe or summer sandal, all are winners. Ballet flats are perfectly apropos as well if you're looking for maximum comfort.

4. A great fitting pair of classic trousers will never steer you wrong. Jeans can be suitable on "Casual Fridays" and in more informal professional environments, if they are a darker wash, not embellished, not too tight and definitely not distressed. Trouser style jeans are a great compromise. Think "appropriateness". If your overall vibe looks like you're about to run errands, you are not dressed properly. However, if you look like a woman who is dressed relaxed but can still be taken seriously, you've probably hit the mark.

5. A sheath dress, shirt dress, wrap or flared dress with a sleeve that hits right around the knee are great options for business casual attire. If your dress has spaghetti straps, you will want to add another layer on top, such as a cropped cardigan or jacket. Avoid mini's, dresses that are so tight that they ride up high on your hips when seated, any dress that looks like a beach cover up, romper styles or a dress that shows too much cleavage. I'm just saying! You're at work after all.

6. Wearing a jacket immediately gives a woman a more polished appearance (whether worn with a skirt, slacks or over a dress). Tank tops, sheer revealing tops, baggy T- shirts, just don't cut it. Do consider more refined looks, like tailored dress shirts, pretty blouses, cardigans, and belted or zippered jackets to channel the powerful woman you are.

7. I have mixed feelings about leggings because so many women abuse this article of clothing, business wear or otherwise. In creative or casual environments, wearing leggings in lieu of tights is acceptable. This looks like a tunic, dress or long cardigan that falls at least mid-thigh paired with leggings and flats or boots. The problems arise when women start wearing leggings as if they are an alternative to pants or jeans. They are most certainly not! I don't care what the label says (jeggings, peggings, yada yada), if a legging or pant is so skin tight on you that we can see when your butt muscles flex, it is not a work-appropriate look. Use common sense. I DO wear leggings when I work with clients, typically in the fall, but I am often pairing these bottoms with knit dresses or very long tunics. Because I am tall and many dresses often fall too short on me, pairing dresses with leggings gives me the flexibility to still wear dresses I like, but be appropriate with it. My rear end is never in play in these ensembles and I recommend that yours is not either.

POLISHED CASUAL DRESS

Many women struggle with looking pulled together in casual settings. They end up under-dressing because they're worried about over dressing. So how do you present a polished and pulled together image while in a casual setting? Here's the short answer: You can still be "dressed" without being "dressed up".

If you're a business woman and you're attending a BBQ where you know you'll meet other business professionals, how do you show up? Do you dress with the baggy T-shirt, shorts and flip flops which, while appropriate for the occasion, may not send that "dressed" signal to those you may want to impress? Or do you show up in a top that flatters you, a pair of well-fitting linen slacks or a cotton skirt, with a jazzy pair of sandals? Both are appropriate for the occasion, both are comfortable. But the latter is infinitely more effective in case you do bump into that person you've been dying to meet and for five minutes you happen to talk business.

I don't know about you, but my policy is to be safe than sorry. More than that, my motto really is this: NOT looking "polished" is never an option. Never an option. Why look "less than" my amazing potential, regardless of the context or situation or environment? I challenge you to ask yourself, why should you?

Be fabulous, regardless of the occasion!

BECOMING *F*ABULOUS

First, determine which of the eight wardrobe-challenged working women scenarios best mirrors your situation. Then, check off the suggestions you are currently implementing and circle ideas you can begin implementing to help get your work gear up to par. Make a to-do list of the new ideas, so that when you plan your next shopping trip, you can narrow down exactly the types of items needed to augment your work wear.

Have your significant other or a friend take photos of you in your work attire each day for a week. You may be horrified to discover that the outfit you swore was your favorite now looks sub-par. This is not unusual. And though you may want to throw in the towel after the first day, keep going. Do this for five days straight and make an honest evaluation of what works and what doesn't. Try to dissect the key style components in each photo: color, fit, pulled togetherness, figure flattery, appropriateness, professionalism, etc.

This is tough to do, but challenge yourself to keep at it. The point is to understand where you need to improve and reinforce the things you are doing that are working. Photos don't lie, so whatever you perceive is wrong about your photos is likely true. If you're unsure, ask a trusted friend for his/her opinion. Let them know they need to be brutally honest with you (and don't get mad at them when you don't like what they say!).

Using the photos as a guide, begin to select different combinations of items already in your closet to start creating more flattering and finished combinations. Take another batch of photos and compare the differences. Repeat as often as you need to. You may need to make a few shopping trips in the interim, to augment your closet with items that will partner more successfully with your clothing. This is all part of the process. The goal is to ultimately land on 5 or 6 FABULOUS work ensembles that you can replicate so you soon have a closet full of business attire that works for you in every way. You'll know you are on the right track when your business associates start complimenting you on the way you look. Rock on!

Chapter Ten

Are you Ready to Flaunt It?

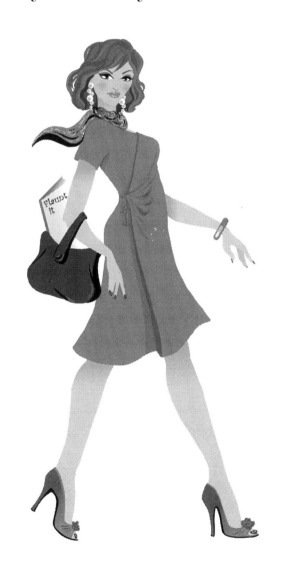

If you've been reading attentively, which I know you have, and putting into practice the advice within these pages, I'm certain you have experienced an upbeat change in attitude, a realization that your image counts, and the joyous feeling that comes from discovering a whole new you blossoming from what was a tiny bud.

When you get right down to it, looking fabulous isn't as much about people's positive reaction to you; it really has a lot to do with how you feel about yourself.

Have you ever noticed how when you put on your favorite outfit, your whole mood lifts? Perhaps you feel sexier and sassier in stockings and high heels? Or maybe you feel more confident and in command when you put on a beautifully tailored suit? Or perhaps you feel positively sensational in your red cocktail dress?

The fact is that clothing really has a psychological impact on how we feel.

The icing on the cake? Your clothing and the way you feel when you wear it, can have a similar psychological impact on those around you. If you feel sexy and sassy, that feeling is almost passed on by osmosis to the people you interact with.

I'm sure you may have experienced it. You are wearing something you know makes you look fabulous, and you sense that fabulousness reflected back at you by others.

That explains why I've spent so much time in this book stressing why the clothing you wear should project the image you want to convey. You start to feel like the person you want to be and then act like that person. Consequently, people perceive you as being that person and respond accordingly.

The clothing you wear has such a profound impact on your image. It actually plays a part in the jobs you get, the relationships you have and your sense of self-esteem. "Dress the part" and you'll start acting the part!

ARE YOU WEARING A 'UNIFORM'?

Some women have to wear uniforms in their daily life. Women in the military live in their uniforms, and many that I've met have never had a reason to think of clothing in terms of style, far less have the know-how to build a closet that works when they're off duty or retired. Many reach out for help with the basics of pulling a look together.

Those who have retired out of the military, typically need more intervention. They have to learn pretty much everything I've been sharing throughout this book to build a wardrobe suitable for their newfound civilian life.

Then there are women who have other types of uniforms. Doctors, pharmacists, scientists, and nurses all wear lab coats or scrubs over their clothing. This becomes a uniform because they could be wearing their pajamas under their coats and we'd be none the wiser. Then there are fields in the technology sector and some service industries that require uniforms.

Women who routinely have a shell over their clothes for work purposes, have a higher likelihood of struggling with their wardrobes because they haven't had to dress to impress. Their lab coats, military or other uniforms become their faces to the world, which communicate the attributes those uniforms are meant to convey. And as the word "uniform" implies, there is nothing individualistic or unique about these outer shells which serve entities or companies, but not an individual with her unique tastes, colors, style and sensibilities. Often, these women's social and casual wardrobes are weak to nonexistent as well, so they wind up lost with no sense of style and resort to another type of "uniform"—their defaults—ensembles that are safe, comfortable or easy.

The good news is if this is you, you are not alone.

To multiply this factor even further, there are many women who do not officially wear a uniform for work or service but who wind up with defaults, regardless. In these instances, a "uniform" could mean wearing the same colors day in day out. Or it could be wearing the same type of skirt suit to work every day. Or it could mean living in jeans, a T-shirt, and running shoes.

These types of "uniforms" do not have to be negative, if the "uniforms" were created with intent, purpose, and serve you. We all have particular silhouettes, designs, colors and ensembles we gravitate towards. Some women do so more than others. But there are two camps. Women who love the uniforms they have created for themselves because they are a reflection of their signature, effortless style, and they feel fabulous. Then there are the women who are sick and tired of their uniforms. These uniforms are their defaults, their go-to's because they don't have the time, skill or inspiration to do differently. The latter often find themselves in a clothing rut because their wardrobes do not reflect their highest, finest vision of themselves.

If you're one of those women who picked up this book because you wanted to spice up your wardrobe and your look, who wanted a variation from her uniform (real or created), this book should have given you many ideas on how to take your look from blah to blazing. My mission is to give you the tools and the confidence to make your true essence shine through your clothing with the advice I've shared in all these chapters. Now *you've* got to put in the work.

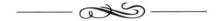

TRANSFORMATION IN ACTION:
MEET BETHANY

Bethany spent 15 years in the US Navy, straight out of high school. Now retired from the military, in her mid-30's and single, she feels completely lost when it comes to clothes and shopping. In fact she avoids shopping at all costs because she winds up overwhelmed and frustrated. Bethany's formative grooming years were spent in a crisp, sharp uniform. In her down time, she resorted to jeans and a Tee or sweatshirt paired with sneakers. She had a few button-down shirts and slacks. However, she didn't own a dress or a skirt that wasn't part of her uniform (even though she had to-die-for legs) because she never had cause to think of her clothing in any way other than functionally.

She came to me before a brief sabbatical, after which she would be transitioning into an executive position at a prominent consulting firm. She was panicked because other than a few interview suits she purchased with the help of a friend, she had no suitable work or social wardrobe for her new life. In addition, Bethany found herself declining the few invitations she received to social events. Because she was insecure about pulling outfits together, she felt awkward and out of place at the few events she did attend. She did not feel she measured up to the other women. So she started declining to venture out altogether. She needed intervention and to get up to speed quickly.

Our work together involved delving into what she wanted her image to project, her goals (professionally and personally), her preferences, lifestyle needs, etc. She had an inverted triangle figure and we worked together on styles and ensembles that enhanced her best features—her long shapely legs and strong shoulder lines. Bethany looked amazing in a pencil skirt and fitted suit jacket. She looked fabulous in halter dresses that hit at the knee. She looked stunning in shift styled dresses paired with a soft cardigan. And I clued her in on the colors that made her shine. By the time she was due to start her new career, she had the basics of a wardrobe in place and a keener sense of the clothing that made her feel great. Bethany's next step is to incorporate accessories into her look to really step up her style game. But now she has the confidence and inspiration to try new things and continue to refine and tweak her style. And she accepts invitations to events so that she can pursue a personal goal of attracting a mate.

Observation: Regardless of her starting point, every woman has the ability to learn the skills and tools to look great. It may mean hiring an image consultant. Regardless of the learning method, the benefits are multifold: A wardrobe that works. A style that reflects who you are. The confidence that comes with looking and feeling great. And for Bethany, the courage to finally feel she could mix with other women without feeling discouraged and estranged. Once she found her style voice, she could start to Flaunt It.

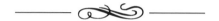

FINDING YOUR EFFORTLESS STYLE

Some of my clients want uniforms, but these are new and improved versions of their old defaults. They want a style that is consistent, that is easy and effortless to pull together and this then becomes their new and vastly improved uniform. Note the huge attitude shift in the notion of uniforms: one originates from apathy, the other from a need for change. Change is good.

One of my clients travels frequently for work and she wanted several ensembles or uniforms she could replicate with ease, to take away the frustration and challenge of figuring out what to pack and wear for a 5-day business trip. For her, style guidelines (uniforms) make sense, because they enable her to dress effortlessly on the road and give her the confidence to know she looks great.

Often at the end of a consultation session, I leave clients with a series of 'Action Items' they need to implement to achieve their image goals. The action can be as simple as finding a new pair of jeans that fit and flatter, to more difficult changes, such as a new hairstyle, or daring to experiment with silhouettes outside their comfort zone. The point is that armed with new knowledge, action is necessary.

The same holds true for you reading these words right now. I don't just want you to read this book and tuck it away on your bookshelf. I want you to embrace the journey and transformation inherent in everything you have learned about your colors, personal style, image goals, figure type, image saboteurs and more. You ARE a new woman from having read this book.

To give you a little nudge, I am going to provide you with a list of 10 really easy things you can implement right now to create a positive change in your look. If you do 3 things, you get a pat on the back. If you do 5, you get a high five. If you do 7 or more, you get The Image Diva's seal of approval and a grade A for taking serious action. Are you ready for this challenge? Here goes!

10 IMAGE/WARDROBE CHANGE AGENTS

1. Scarves are an easy and chic enhancer to many looks. They come in all colors, varieties, textures and styles. Easy breezy and effortless. There are very feminine lacy styles that are perfect for warmer temps that add instant style to your ensembles. If you prefer traditional scarves, then opt for one in a bright color that complements you.

2. Speaking of colors—this is an effortless way to change how you look and feel. Wear colors that make you radiate, make your eyes sparkle and make your skin glow. You'll know you're on the right track because you're sure to get compliments. Just changing the colors of your tops and jackets can be an immediate image boost and one that people immediately notice. Know your "wow" colors and start wearing them.

3. Every woman needs that great fitting pair of jeans. I recently took 6 women shopping and it is very difficult to find the perfect pair of jeans in one trip. There are SO many factors that go into finding the perfect pair of jeans, I devoted an entire section of the book to that. Go back to chapter 6, review, and then go shopping. Once you find *your* pair, you will feel like a new woman, I assure you.

4. Invest in a great haircut or new style. Nothing gives a woman an instant boost more than her crowning glory—her hair. Whether you decide to change the color, style or get augments—just make sure the result is realistic to maintain

and in sync with your personal or professional image goals. There are great sites that let you virtually try on hair, so do use the Internet as a resource to experiment first. Make sure you have a good rapport with your stylist because you are essentially putting your hair in their hands.

5. Cardigans have become ubiquitous and are the epitome of effortless chic. They come in a variety of colors, lengths and styles. I am not so crazy about the really long styles with the peaked edges, because I think they shorten the legs of most women. But I do like the waist length cardigan (for those days when you need another layer for warmth and still want to look cute) or the hip length cardigan which is oh so great for cinching with skinnier belts. The more flattering designs, contour to the body so they look great belted or can be worn unbuttoned over your favorite top. Don't feel obligated to button all the buttons. A neat trick is to start buttoning from the third or fourth button down and leave the last button undone as well.

6. Try adding one new makeup application to your regimen. You'd be surprised at the boost that can give your face. Maybe it is finally daring to wear red-toned lipstick. Or it may be a new eye shadow color. For me recently, it was discovering this amazing eyeliner that did not run. I can finally line my lower lids again without worrying I'll look like a raccoon in an hour. And that makes a difference in how my eyes look. So it can be a subtle change or a bigger one, but the point is it will help in making your face a focal point.

7. I am a big fan of women looking like women, which means I love to see the contours and silhouette of the feminine form, and a big part of that is the waist. I often encourage my clients to cinch their waists if it makes sense, given their body, proportions and preferences. Belts are a wonderful accessory to have in your collection for this purpose. If you're not fond of belts, look for waist cinching designs like ruching, contouring, wrap styles or corseting. These all will help give you that hourglass silhouette most of us admire.

8. Start paying attention to your posture. So many of us walk, sit and stand with a slouch or slump to our shoulders and back. One of the things that immediately gives a woman presence and a look of confidence is a straight strong shoulder line. If you are blessed with shoulders balanced to your hips, take advantage of the blessing. Standing erect not only makes you look poised, but also slimmer and taller. For women with narrow shoulders, look for details in tops that extend the shoulder line, such as a boat neck collar, shoulder pads, puffed

sleeves, etc. Having poise gives you presence and ensures that people take no-tice of you in a crowd.

9. I am a big believer in getting all the help I can to ensure I look fabulous in my clothing. Foundation garments, ladies! This includes your bra. Make sure your bra lifts and supports the girls. If you're small busted like me, a push-up, padded bra can create instant cleavage. Trust me. For those with extra softness around the tummy, hips and rear, shapewear can be your best friend. There are many styles and brands available. Find the one that does the trick for you.

10. Last but not least. When did you last shop your own closet? What does that mean? It means treating your closet like a treasure trove where you discover new finds and new ways to combine, layer and coordinate items. You will be surprised at how many items you have sitting in your closet right now, that are just dying to be paired with another friend that's also sitting lonely in your closet. I remember doing a closet audit for a client where I showed her two new ways to wear a bustier she had. We paired the bustier with a collared shirt under it for one look and for the second look, we layered the bustier with a jacket in her closet. And of course she could wear the bustier as a stand alone item. There are countless examples of this, right in your own closet. Take a few hours one weekend and just have fun playing in your wardrobe. Look for new and interesting ways to create new outfits and make a list of what you are missing for the next time you go shopping.

PURGING FOR PANACHE

Now that you've begun the transformation into a new, brighter and bolder "you", what will you do differently? A critical part of refining your style so you are able to Flaunt It, is assessing your wardrobe to find out which items enhance your image and which ones don't and need to be discarded. Clothing which no longer serves you or is no longer relevant to your life and lifestyle, has to go. It's tossing out time ladies!

Sure, this is tough because there may well be items you still love, but you've got to be ruthless and start purging. It is only when you can really see the clothing you own that flatters, fits, and enhances you, that you can take the steps to rebuild a wardrobe that works for you and that reflects you, so dressing becomes effortless. I promise it will ultimately make you feel a whole lot better in the long run.

Pick a day to dedicate to purging your closet. Get 3 boxes, containers or large bags so that you can create 3 categories of clothing that will move out of your closet:

- Menders

- Giveaways

- Throw aways

The final category, **Keepers**, will be clothes that will be left hanging in your closet after your purge. **Keepers** are those items that are relevant for your new image and those that fit, flatter and enhance your figure. These are clothes you love that are also in sync with your new, fab vision for yourself.

Let's go through the other 3 categories:

Menders may simply need slight alterations or tailoring to make them work for you. A hem up or down, a taking in here and there, just minor tweaks a skilled tailor can perform to make the item look amazing on you. If the item is old and needs major overhauling, it's probably best to toss it in the "Throw away" pile.

Giveaways are items of clothing that are still in good shape, but no longer fit you (literally and metaphorically). Now that you know what works for you, these items may be the wrong color, cut or style so they need to move on to another life. Or perhaps they are items you never wore for one reason or another and they are taking up valuable closet real estate. Time to discard them. Giving these items to a local refuge or women's shelter will make you feel good about yourself too.

Throw aways are items that have outlived their shelf life. You'll know instinctively which ones these are, but you may have trouble parting with them. It is hard to get rid of any item that may have sentimental value or strong emotional associations for you. This is where engaging the help of a trusted friend comes in handy. Let her be ruthless. Remind yourself "out with the old, in with the new" as in the new *you*. Toss any item that is old, dated, tattered, stained, worn out and otherwise unwearable.

When you're done, have a good, honest look at what is left. Does your closet look more like the woman you are aspiring to be? What would help make it more versatile? What are you missing that could help pull your looks together? Maybe it's a few more good quality foundation garments, or a couple of layering pieces like Tee's and camis.

Or it could be something you've never considered (or have considered, but not been brave enough to purchase!) like a signature handbag or brighter colored pieces.

Once you've assessed the gaps in your wardrobe, the fun part is going shopping to add those missing pieces to your closet. If you've taken note of all the advice in this book, shopping will be a fantastic opportunity to really invest in pieces that make a statement about who you are.

Perhaps as you examine your newly purged closet, you can observe that the skirt you've worn with the same jacket for the past 5 years would look incredible with the silk emerald green top you've been trying to find a partner for? Ahh... yes the thrill of creating new looks with clothes you've always owned. When you start to really *see* your clothes in a new light, you will be empowered to experiment with different looks and combinations. There is something wonderfully liberating about that, my friend.

Now is the time to venture into uncharted territory. If you've read this far, you are ready for it!

Change is a constant in our life, but it can be challenging to cope with too much change too quickly. If you need to start your transformation with baby steps, that's okay. If you are a "list maker", get out your journal and list all the new additions you intend making to your wardrobe and then tick them off as you purchase each one.

EVERY OCCASION IS AN OPPORTUNITY TO FLAUNT IT

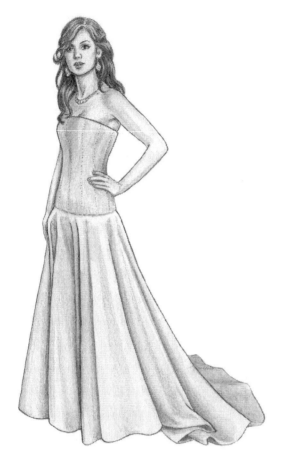

Your wardrobe is a mirror reflecting the woman you present to the world. If you aspire to be perceived as successful, then your wardrobe should be outfitted with items befitting the power broker that you are.

Every occasion, no matter how casual or formal, is an opportunity to Flaunt your signature style. Use the advice and guidelines in this book to help you select outfits that turns heads and conveys the image you want to Flaunt.

Let's have a look at a range of social and professional occasions where you can dress to impress.

❖ For office parties, you want to be more conservative than other events, while still looking festive. Avoid provocative necklines and ultra short skirts unless you want to be the focus of office gossip around the water cooler for the next 12 months. Separates are always a good choice; a crisp, white ruffled blouse paired with an elegantly tailored skirt or black pants is a sophisticated and feminine look, while being very office appropriate. Give your ensemble some zing with bold accessories.

❖ Holiday parties are the ideal occasions to let your hair down and express your signature style. They are the perfect event to really go to town. For the woman who wants to stand out and be noticed, look for a dress that boldly says, "Let's party!" How? Fun and flirty details, vivid colors, shorter length, interesting details like tiers, fringe or faux fur, all can do the trick. Want to look fashion-forward and alluring? Dazzle in a sleeveless number. Add a saucy leather shrug or pashmina for pizzazz.

❖ Who says black tie has to mean a black dress? Wear any color that makes you look and feel fabulous—the bolder, the better! Festive events call for festive colors, so think about fire engine red, teal, chartreuse, gun metal grey, rich emerald, lustrous gold or whatever color takes your fashion fancy. Look for rich, polished fabrics that convey sophistication and elegance such as silk, satin, taffeta, velvet and chiffon. Tulle used as an underskirt or for embellishment is an exquisite detail. For a sophisticated and edgy look, opt for a fitted tuxedo jacket with silk, leather or satin lapels teamed with a pair of tapered black pants or full legged slacks. Add a sexy, sparkly cami or French lace bustier to turn heads.

❖ Working out? When you wear clothes that flatter your body shape, you feel better about yourself and more motivated during your workout. Better yet, if you have an array of cute, comfortable and flattering workout wear to choose from, you'll be more excited about getting dressed to get to the gym and more motivated to keep up your workout regime.

❖ Travel in comfort and style by choosing outfits that are easy to wear, practical and comfortable, without looking as though you just got out of bed. Take the time to plan your travel wardrobe so you have as many variations as possible by mixing and matching ensembles and accessories.

❖ Pregnancy is no excuse not to look fabulous. Once upon a time pregnancy used to be an excuse to let it all hang out—literally. Nine months of not worrying about tucking in your tummy, wearing high heels or looking fabulous. Whoa! A big thank you has to go to the plethora of celebs who have shown us that being pregnant is no excuse for not looking radiant and stunning. Proudly Flaunt your baby bump by wearing styles, prints and colors that work with your newfound figure and radiance, and get out there and glow! Prints, maxi dresses, empire waisted tops and dresses, and the creative use of layering, are all techniques you can use to look beautiful while pregnant.

TO FLAUNT

Once you've discovered your style, and you're feeling fabulicious, how do you begin to Flaunt It and what does that even mean? The dictionary defines the verb 'to Flaunt' as follows: *"to parade or display oneself conspicuously, defiantly, or boldly."* Wow!

Quite the attitude, huh? But isn't this the hallmark of confidence? To boldly strut and let the world know you've got it?

There are varying degrees of Flaunting and this book certainly is not meant to turn you into an obnoxious you-know-what. Rather, it is to urge you to "own" your fabulousness. To step into your brilliance proudly and let others see your magnificence shining from the inside out.

So what does a woman who Flaunts It look like?

She looks great and she knows it. She embraces who she is and what she stands for. Her inner core and outward presentation are perfectly aligned. She is acutely aware of her personal style and executes it every day, every time—consistently. She gets it. She understands the power inherent in having an image that is a notch above.

If you want to be perceived as such a woman, read these seven tips for even more guidance.

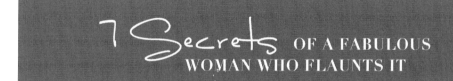

1. **Strengthen your Inner Core**
   No I'm not talking about your muscles here. Flaunting It requires confidence, self-possession and complete comfort in your own skin. Remember you can only reflect outward what you believe about yourself. Continue to work on your self-image and self-esteem so these are no longer barriers to looking great. When you can be fearless about how you approach life, when others' opinions and perceptions do not define you, and when your inner beauty is aligned with what is seen on the outside, THEN you will effortlessly Flaunt It.

2. **Have a Defined Signature Style**
   Know your signature style. The way you express yourself via your clothing is your advertisement about who you are and what you stand for. What *do* you stand for? Regardless, it must be credible, authentic, sustainable and consistent.

3. **Utilize Experts**

   Be clear about the limits of your own knowledge. Women who look fabulous don't wing it. They don't leave their appearance to chance. They often hire experts to perfect their image and mold a personal style that is unforgettable. Some invest in stylists, image consultants, or personal shoppers for assistance, so that looking fabulous becomes truly effortless.

4. **Be Organized**

   An organized closet is one that is easy to work with. You see everything and clothing is organized by color, function, or design and you can mix and match with aplomb. A well-ordered closet is key to creating polished, effortless ensembles and avoiding unnecessary wardrobe duplication.

5. **Have outfits for every Occasion**

   Women who Flaunt It own a well-rounded wardrobe that mirrors their lifestyles, personal styles, personalities and goals. So whether it's a board meeting or a fundraiser, they always have the right outfits to shine.

6. **Timelessness not Trendiness**

   Smart women focus on style and its impact, not fashion trends. They care less about trends and invest in clothing uniquely appointed to complement their image goals, figure and personal brand. They ensure they invest in timeless pieces that fit impeccably.

7. **Be a Woman of Consequence**

   A woman of consequence is a woman with a purpose. She has a life and she is busy living it. She knows who she is and what she wants to achieve. She uses her image as a tool to facilitate her success in all areas of her life. She Flaunts It because she can. We believe her because she sure as heck believes in herself. "To thine own self be true" is a principle she takes to heart.

I want to talk to you for a moment about the transformation that results when a woman takes the time to refine, revamp or revitalize her image.

For a lucky minority, it can happen very quickly if they are primed and ready to take action to achieve quick and life changing results. For some women, transformation is slower, more paced, more trial and error, but successful nonetheless. Still other women need multiple reinforcement to make it 'click'; for all the pieces to come together before they start to see the results they seek. This is probably true for the majority of women. For the rest, it is a lifelong refinement, a continual tweaking, an ongoing quest and desire to shine as brightly as possible.

I have a special passion for the ladies who recognize the value in investing in themselves and continually seek to elevate their style game. Some of the most fabulous women I know fall into this category, me included.

The point is, the journey is unique and individual to each woman, pretty much like in life. Our journeys to self-acceptance and actualization are as unique as we all are and I want you to take a moment to acknowledge and celebrate THAT!

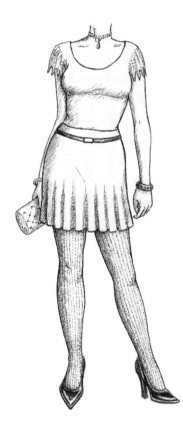

An image refinement is the ultimate gift that keeps on giving. It brings me no greater fulfillment than to see women evolve in their style sensibilities and to push the boundaries of what they before perceived to be the limits of their beauty. The transformations can be 'quiet' or on full broadcast. But regardless, each woman is renewed with a sense of confidence and emboldened to express her very best expression to others. Wherever you are on your own journey, be present, be authentic and really go for it. Reach for the stars and push yourself to be as brilliant as you can. If we collectively take this approach, think of all the twinkling, shining, magnificence that we'll all manifest.

Again we come back to my personal mantra, "Presence with a Purpose"™. By practicing intent in every aspect of your appearance, you present the best possible image to the world; a powerful, purposeful and *effective* image that is magnetic. One that projects a cool, confident persona that clearly says, "This woman has effortless style. She looks fabulous, and boy is she Flaunting It!"

A FEW PARTING WORDS

This quote was shared with me by my yoga teacher Heffer. It sums up more beautifully than I can ever articulate, why the world needs to see you in your highest and finest vision of yourself, at all times.

> "There is a vitality, a life force, an energy, a quickening that is translated through you into action. And because there is only one of you in all of time, this expression is unique. And if you block it, it will never exist through any other medium; the world will not have it. It is not your business to determine how good it is, nor how valuable, nor how it compares with other expressions. It is your business to keep it yours clearly and directly, to keep the channel open."
> **– Martha Graham, The Expression of You**

It has been my absolute pleasure to write this book and fill you with inspiration, motivation, and encouragement and arm you with knowledge. Thank you so much for letting me share my expertise with you. It will absolutely facilitate your image transformation, if you embrace the process.

Remember that you are not alone in your struggles and frustrations. We've all experienced similar challenges at one point or another. But with the advice, secrets and tips I have shared on these pages, you now have an advantage—the know-how to dress and present the image of your choosing, one created with intent and designed by you. Your revamped image can become the inspiration for another woman to get her act together. Isn't that amazing?

If you've stayed with me this whole time, you have already begun your transformation into a new more fabulous you. Your journey has already begun.

Congratulations!!

If this book has transformed your life, share the gift with others. Gift the book to the beloved women in your life so they too can experience their own unique journey from frumpy to fabulous!

Here's to looking Fabulous and Flaunting It!

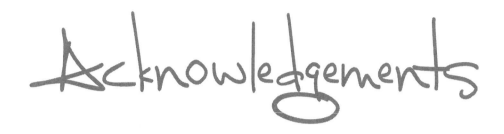

Acknowledgements

This book would not be possible without the tremendous support, advice and teamwork from trusted friends, colleagues and professionals. Thank you so much for making my dream a reality!

Special thanks to the following wonderful spirits:

Heffer—My spiritual guide. Your humility and wisdom inspire and enlighten me. I've grown so much by your teachings over the years. You have helped me express my finest, highest version of myself by tapping into my Source. I am a better human "being" for having known you!

Ros O—You were there at the beginning helping me to create a structure for my myriad ideas. Thank you for creating the template –I could not have done this on my own. I appreciate how accommodating you were and just plain 'ole fun. You took an overwhelming task and made it manageable and never complained. Thank you!

Mia R—You have and continue to be the voice of reason and caution. You taught me so much by example and by mentoring. You dared me to see the big picture and the ultimate vision. That counsel has been priceless. Thank you for believing in my limitless potential. Your referrals to resources for this book was so needed –thank you for sharing them with me. You are amazing! Thank you for being an inspiration to me. I am forever grateful for all your advice throughout the course of this book project and I'm humbled by the generosity of your time with me.

Clare A—Thank you for your genuine excitement about this project. You were among the first few people I told. Your advice about the cover was perfectly timed. You may not know it, but your counsel early on gave me much needed encouragement to know I could do this. And I did!

Ann Catherine—You are SO talented. Your illustrations bring my book to life. You are a delight to work with always!

Maryam H—You got the gist of the image I wanted for my cover with just a few e-mail exchanges. You rock!! Thank you for my sassy Diva who is most certainly Flaunting It.

Carolyn S—How long does it take to complete a book? Forever apparently, when I'm at the helm. You have been beyond patient and accommodating. I am so grateful that I chose you to design my book. I had NO idea that I could let it drag on as long as I did. Thank you for being you—always supportive, flexible and so insanely patient. Thank you so much! You did a great job!

Tim T—You are always patient, forever rooting for me. Your advice, support and friendship means so much to me. Thank you for taking time to share your point of view on this book every time I asked for it.

Maurice M, Larry C, Trevor C—You are such good friends. You always have great ideas and I can always count on your support, whatever my endeavor. Thank you for your creative ideas and always positive attitude.

To my inner circle of "advisers" who each helped make this book a better product for their contribution and support at varying stages: Traci N, Lara A, Jeff S, Sandra B, Tammy H, Leroy M, Monique L, Antoinette K and Adrian M. Thank you guys!!

Cousin Kenneth—You always allow me to dream big and you listen. Thanks for always thinking I can!

Kenneth Clapp photography—That was my most fun photo shoot ever! Thank you for helping me show my readers how I Flaunt It! Thank you for helping me bring out my *sparkle*.

To my family, especially my 3 young nephews (who have no interest in the content of this book, incidentally) who I hope will be inspired to pursue their own dreams accordingly, when they come of age.

Last but not least I want to thank my clients who are my ultimate inspiration. I am so privileged to have played a part in each of your unique image journeys. Collectively you have allowed me to give, inform and empower on topics that I am so deeply passionate about. Most of all, you made my mission very clear. Because of you I saw a need that I felt compelled to share with the millions more that could benefit from my expertise. This book is part of my legacy and one of the ways to support my platform: "Mission 1 Million Makeovers: Change Your Image, Transform your Life." This is just the beginning. Thank you for your support. Thank you, Thank you, Thank you!

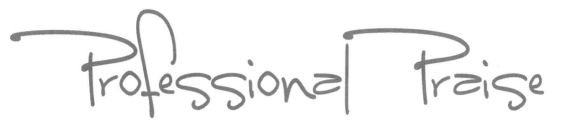

Professional Praise

"[Natalie] is really something special, she seems motivated by making us all feel BETTER about how we look. I am so used to berating myself with that voice in my head which picks on things I don't like about my looks, shape, or wardrobe. Natalie drowns out that voice by empowering women to embrace who they are—as they are—and making every shape, size, age, etc. look and feel GREAT." —Tracy

"I am very thankful for having found you. In a very short period of time, your way of explaining what and why combined with your compassion for when I was nervous about a new direction really helped me know that I COULD change the way I look for the better. And not just in one outfit, but throughout my entire wardrobe.

Spending time with you taught me that I can easily dress in a way that reflects who I truly am (all facets of me—not just one or two) and look great! Also, that I can stop being overwhelmed when I go shopping and I can find clothes that look great on me (that aren't just black and white).

I can't tell you how grateful I am. You have truly helped me (quickly) through this part of integrating myself into a more whole, beautiful being—inside and out! Thank you very much.

Lastly, your ability to "keep it simple" is helping me to remember what to do for myself and to try new combinations in my existing wardrobe—everyday. I even did it this morning and I feel great today." —Teresa

"(Natalie) knocked my socks off. I cannot recommend her highly enough. I enjoyed our time immensely and felt terrific after our meeting. I promise you, you will not be disappointed and will feel invigorated to make positive changes in your wardrobe which will make you feel better inside too." —Vicky

"I always get compliments now, thanks to you and Elan! I love it-it's such a boost." —Anne

"My day with Natalie learning about how the way I dress and carry myself is a day I will never forget. Being a senior in high school and still trying to figure out who I am is a journey, which is why it is important to dress the way I want others to perceive me. Natalie is such a sincere person but also told me what was good and what was bad, even if it wasn't quite what I wanted to hear. (No purple prom dress for me) On the other hand, she worked with me to find the colors that don't just make me look good, but make me look the best! I can't thank you enough for what you have taught me, not only about the colors I choose and the accessories I wear, but by showing confidence, you can go along way." —Moira

"I can't tell you how happy I am about my purchases. Having you with me gave me the confidence to know I was choosing great items and I feel like they all fill gaps in my wardrobe. I am thrilled!" —Cindy

"The transformational aspect of the session for me was the huge leap in my under-standing of all the little decisions and non-decisions that have a big effect on how I am perceived by others.

I went through a period of time when I took so many of those decisions for granted largely out of the mindset that all that really matters is my ability to think and do work. I couldn't have cared any less about winning style points.

One thing that you said that really sunk in deeply with me is making the shift from approaching others to being approached by others, personally and professionally. When I have achieved that, I will know the transformation has absolutely happened!"
—Darien

"Everything was informative! I do very much appreciate at the end the "image statement" that was put together at the end of the session. Those words pop up in my mind whenever I shop for clothes, or wherever I go. They reinforce my resolve and decisive action about conveying the image I want, and a sense of accomplishment for investing in my well being. This stuff is like therapy! This was an excellent experience. You're given the tools you need to move forward intentionally and positively. My first time out shopping was completely different because of how I applied the knowledge I had gained, and boy did I get compliments!" —Valerie

"Thank you so much for the wonderful workshop on Saturday. I was truly inspired afterwards, and even went to Nordstroms over the weekend—I did not feel nearly as helpless and lost as I usually do while shopping :) I even got a couple pair of summer shoes that I actually love (!), and I got a pair of NYDJ that they are tailoring this week! Now at least I have 2 items from your list of must-haves…a big improvement for me! I am looking forward to working with you again in the future."
—Alice

"Thank YOU. You bring a wonderful spirit and enthusiasm to this—and as a result, I enjoyed every moment of it. Today I wore the long jacket we bought with the trimmest black pants I have, and got a million compliments. So, great success…I confess to taking one thing out of the throwaway pile –but everything else is gone!! And, your suggestions in this email are wonderful. I will try them all. Thanks so very much."
—Judy

"Let's talk awesome colors and feeling fun, happy and confident in colors that say what you FEEL. Thank you Natalie for showing me how to use color to express myself in my clothing and create the attitude about my appearance that I want to project using complimentary colors. My session for personal color consultation was time and money well spent! Personal style takes form on many different levels—but for me (thanks to expert Elan advice), my style has taken a quantum leap forward recently as a result of color consultation. LADIES, I HIGHLY RECOMMEND THIS to everyone. I am a believer! So much so that I plan to have the service done for my daughter as a gift. Talk to Natalie...SERIOUSLY...do this." —Susi D

"Natalie is an inspiration, she took a much needed area for teen girls and turned into a fun and educational day!" —Susan

"I was very pleased with my image consultation with Natalie. As soon as I walked through her doors, I felt that she could almost read my persona. We talked extensively, discussing what my needs, wants and my way ahead would be. She was very detailed in discussing what works and what does not work.

Example: I'm encouraged to no longer wear running shoes, blue jeans and baggy t-shirts as an outing outfit...actually her words were, "...you're not allowed to wear running shoes unless you're going running". However, she didn't stop there...she continued to show me alternatives to a casual, comfortable look that had polish and style without much fuss. I've historically been a blue jean and T-shirt kind of gal. Additionally I'm an Army service member who wears a uniform everyday...and have been fashion challenged for some time. Natalie provided me tools, great professional advice and was sincere and honest in our discussions. I'm going to embark on my first shopping experience armed with my new tools this weekend and I feel empowered and confident that I can accomplish my goals." —Maureen

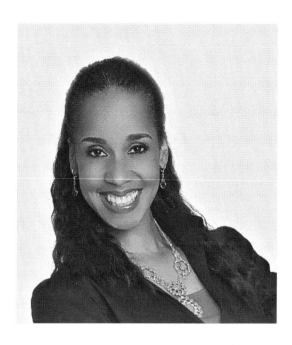

About the Author

Natalie Jobity, President of Elan Image Management, and founder of "Mission 1 Million Makeovers: Change your Image, Transform your Life" is a sought after image consultant who works with women to help them define and project their unique signature style and an image that positions them for success in all areas of their lives. Her foundational belief is that image refinement can be a facilitator for inward change and growth and vice versa. From this approach, she sees herself as a transformation agent, using image, fashion and wardrobe as the vehicles of change.

Natalie has been featured in a variety of print and online publications locally and nationally as an image expert and has been interviewed several times for television. She has worked with a diverse clientele: Judges, Lawyers, Doctors, women in the Military, Entrepreneurs, Executives, Moms, Coaches, Artists, Teens and others. She was one of the women profiled in the compilation by Andrea Howe, *"Hear Us Roar! 28 Stories of Everyday Women Leading Extraordinary Lives"* whose proceeds benefits charities nationwide.

Natalie routinely speaks on image-related topics to women's groups, organizations and associations. She was born and raised in Trinidad & Tobago and currently resides in the DC metro area.

For media inquiries, contact Elan@ElanImageManagement.com

For more information on Natalie's work
as an image consultant, visit:
www.ElanImageManagement.com.

Share your Image Transformation stories!
Join our community of women and learn more about
"Mission 1 Million Makeovers:
Change Your Image, Transform your Life" ™.
Visit: www.1millionmakeovers.com.

Made in the USA
Lexington, KY
09 April 2012